No Regrets
(Well maybe just a few)

*An intimate reflection of a troubled soul
in search of love (sort of)*

Jenny Webster

Copyright © 2021 by Jenny Webster

All rights reserved. No part of this book may be reproduced or used in any manner without written permission of the copyright owner except for the use of quotations in a book review.

ISBNs:
Paperback: 978-1-80227-101-0
eBook: 978-1-80227-102-7

The names in this book have been changed to protect the not-so innocent. And I have decided to change mine, at least for the time being, as I am not so sure I want my children reading about some of the dodgy choices I made and the brief encounters I had following my divorce. Having said that, my children are not stupid and probably have a really good idea of what I actually got up to. Ce la vie.

No regrets-

I read a couple of quotes which resonated with me before I wrote this book.

"The struggles we endure today will be the "good old days" we laugh about tomorrow. (Aaron Lauritsen)

I certainly have had a laugh about a few of my struggles, but not all of them, so I thought if I can't laugh about them at least I can write about them

Another quote I quite like by Lemmy Kilmister is the following "I don't do regrets. Regrets are pointless. It's too late for regrets. You've already done it, haven't you? You've lived your life. No point wishing you could change it."

How very true. And as I have probably lived at least half of my life already and I definitely can't change what I've done, all I can do is look back at it and smile, and perhaps try to be a better person moving forward.

Contents

Preface   vii

Chapter 1   The curse of bad skin   1

Chapter 2   The curse of anorexia   9

Chapter 3   The curse of bulimia   17

Chapter 4   Off to London   23

Chapter 5   Beauty is supposed to be in the eye of the beholder…   43

Chapter 6   Leading up to and including my marriage   64

Chapter 7   Bucket lists   76

Chapter 8   Internet dating   87

Chapter 9   A Happy Ending?   164

Preface

I first started to think about writing this book when I met my current partner, which sounds a little odd as there is quite a lot about other men in it. But meeting my partner felt like a new beginning for me, following years of mixed up feelings. Feelings about my sense of self-worth. Feelings about my inadequacies and always the need to try to be that perfect woman, perfect wife, perfect mother, with perfect skin and a perfect smile. And when I started to think about everything I had been through I wondered how many women have shared, or continue to have, similar experiences.

There might be some stuff in this book that you can relate to and maybe some stuff that will make you laugh a little. I hope some women who read this book might identify to some extent with my journey and perhaps in some small way it might even help them, or simply make them smile should they relate to some of my experiences.

My eldest daughter actually encouraged me to write this book. She has cried and laughed with me so much over the years and continues to have absolute faith in my ability to get through whatever challenges come my way. Her complete steadfast support and loyalty combined with a huge innate kindness never ceases to amaze me. Without her I probably would have crumbled.

From my experience it definitely really helps to have someone you can confide in. Someone you can be totally honest with. And it certainly helps to have someone you can phone at two am in the morning when you are completely pissed and missed your last train home yet again, lost your purse and need help. My daughter very often was that friend.

Life is full of curved balls and in many ways I have been incredibly lucky. I have never suffered a major illness, I haven't had a major accident, I haven't experienced any real suffering (although trust me, itchy and weeping folliculitis around your fanny isn't too pleasant), I have three incredible children and have travelled to some amazing places. I hope this book will appeal to women who perhaps are relatively "normal" whatever that means and will enjoy reading some of the relatively stupid crazy things I have done, most of which I don't regret, including the two Italians, and I am still here to tell the tale. I guess it could have all ended in tears but thankfully the tears I have now are usually because I am laughing too hard or watching a silly, soppy movie. I really am so lucky.

The second half of this book will contain quite a lot of references to various parts of the anatomy, and in particular vaginas and penises. I was trying to decide what were the best names for these intimate parts of our body and after some consideration decided, moving forward, to use 'fanny' and 'cock', as these seem the most inoffensive names I can think of. I did actually write down a list of all the names I could think of before going with fanny and cock:

Vagina- vag, mini, front bottom (god I hate that one), fru, pussy, twat, slit (yuk), flower, mons, scabbard???, beaver, cooter, fish lips (please no), muff, fuck hole, quim, pounani - I could go on and on ...

Penis, prick, dick, whang, weeny (def had a few of these), member, rod, knob, love muscle, shaft, trouser snake, one-eyed monster, King Dong (not as good as it sounds), Tiny Tim (equally disappointing), Tadger, Old boy and on and on and on.

I think I should just mention that this book definitely isn't an advice book or some grand lecture on conquering the impossible. I do hope it will be fun to read and maybe some of it will strike a chord with you. And who knows, perhaps like me, you will one day meet your perfect partner on a dating website.

Chapter 1

The curse of bad skin

Whilst my upbringing and younger life was in no way extra special or particularly difficult, we all can agree that the experiences we have in younger life in some way have a greater or lesser effect on the choices we make in our future Apparently I was an "accident". Youngest of three, conceived by mistake but nevertheless loved equally by my parents. I was quite clever, and irritatingly "always right" according to mum. I passed the eleven plus, but refused to go to the local grammar school as I said they were all a bunch of snobs (all three of my own children passed the test and went to grammar schools so I am a total hypocrite).

I did the usual amount of skiving and tried to be popular, even though I wasn't. Too frumpy and not pretty enough. I got bullied a bit, although I am sure many of us have, and despite this did surprisingly well in my exams.

Once I started secondary school my life changed. Not because of all the usual pressures that boys and girls go through when they start secondary school, but it was because of what happened when I went through puberty at around the age of twelve. It was then that I started to develop spots. This combined with rather thin and lanky hair made me very self-conscious. And we weren't allowed to wear makeup at school which made things so much worse for me. I remember getting some concealer and a mascara confiscated one day and I was, literally, beside myself. Concealer to me was, and still is, one of the most important possessions I own and I literally will not go anywhere without it even though I may not have to get it out of my bag to use it so much these days. There is something inside most people that leads them to think it's OK to make judgements about others who have spots. As if acne is somehow the fault of the person who has it. Spotty teenagers, or adults for that matter, do not wash enough or eat too much chocolate or don't look after themselves.

And bad skin is ugly. No-one with bad skin gets good jobs or becomes famous. When is the last time you saw someone on TV that has a face full of spots? And how many times do women get criticized on TV for wearing too much makeup, and yet maybe they needed it to give them confidence. People can be so unkind. One of the biggest things that has impacted me in my life, which probably seems pathetic to many people, is in fact the state of my skin. I was probably about thirteen when my skin really started to get bad and it was then that I developed severe acne. I honestly think the state of my skin has impacted on just about everything I have ever done in my life up until now. The self-loathing and utter despair that having bad skin caused me simply cannot be underestimated. I truly think it is impossible to understand the effect bad skin has on a person unless you have had it yourself. It really took me till I was in my mid 50s before I had some treatment that worked, and that finally means I don't wake up in the morning dreading what my skin will look like in the mirror. Having said that I am now fighting a losing battle against the inevitable wrinkles and still have pores the size of small potholes.

When I think about how many potions I have bought and how many treatments I have had to try to improve the look of my skin I am quite frankly embarrassed and disgusted with myself. How can I be that vain and that stupid? I could have probably bought a small semi-detached house for all the money I have wasted. And what is even more sad is the way my emotions have been meddled with. The feeling of hope as I try something new out that promises to cure acne, reduce the size of pores and even out the skin tone, only to be disappointed yet again at the failure to notice any difference in my skin at all. And as I write this the doorbell has just rung and Amazon have delivered a small package containing a bottle of Peptide Complex Serum which might help my wrinkles, so it seems I will never learn.

My mother did try to help me "improve" the condition of my skin. And I have continued to try to "improve" the state of my skin for all of my adult life. We tried facial steaming where I would put my head over a bowl of extremely hot water with a towel put over my head. After about twenty minutes I would come up for some air before plunging my face in a sink of freezing cold water. My face was so red after this that for a minute I thought it looked better as the red spots were somehow less obvious, but actually it really just seemed to bring out more spots. I tried this cream called Eskamel – a really smelly, so called skin-colour cream that dries out after about five minutes. I have no idea if this stuff is still available, but seriously do not try it as it really doesn't do anything. I also tried another strange green coloured cream, designed to make the skin look less red- but this just seemed to make mine look more oily and extremely weird.

I tried all sorts of face masks designed to cleanse, bring out the impurities, dry up excess oil and balance the skin. Mum came up with all sorts of home cures and we tried egg whites, lemon juice, bicarbonate of soda, TCP, toothpaste and many more

I went on various types of antibiotics which helped a little and different contraceptive pills which were supposed to help, but nothing really ever fixed the problem.

I blamed what I was eating, how much water I was drinking, how much sleep I was getting, how fat I was, how thin I was; in fact I hated myself so much and secretly cried so much behind closed doors. If you saw someone on a bus who had no hair, you would probably think they had cancer and feel incredibly sorry for them. If you saw a woman with acne all over her face you would probably turn away. At one point I wished I could have cancer instead of bad skin as at least there might be a chance I would recover from cancer, but I could never see an end to having bad skin, and I just found it unbearable.

One of the issues I faced on a daily basis with spots was whether to squeeze or not to squeeze. Some of you who are reading this book, may in their youth perhaps have had this dilemma? The problem is that if you have a ripe whitehead, the urge to squeeze it is simply irresistible and every time you catch sight of the spot in a mirror it seems to be looking back at you. Goading you. Inviting you to touch it, to squeeze it. You find yourself having no control over what you do and as soon as you get a moment in private you simply just have to give it a squeeze. Sadly the orgasmic ooh and satisfaction you get for a nano-second as the puss squirts out soon fades in to self-hatred for not leaving your skin alone and probably making it worse. Getting blackheads out of blocked pores also seems momentarily satisfying, but then you are left with huge pore holes that no amount of foundation or make-up can ever possibly cover up.

The worst spots are those that don't have a head on them and that sit underneath your skin; a painful lump that you just cannot help but touch, even though you know it will all end in tears. You try wrapping some toilet paper around your fingers to supposedly stop the skin breaking, you start gently, massaging the lump with your fingers but still nothing comes out and the spot remains defiant, just looking more swollen and much redder. You begin to sweat and panic thinking maybe if I stick a needle in it there will be a way for the puss to erupt from. But still nothing happens as you squeeze harder and harder until you completely break the skin and now things are much worse. The lump is still there but now there is also a weeping scarred face that is going to take ages to heal, and you know putting makeup on it will be almost impossible.

"Oh why, oh why did I do that? I am such an idiot. I am so pathetic. I fucking hate myself. God I'm revolting. What the hell am I going to do? I can't go out looking like this. Shit, everyone will look at me. I fucking hate, hate, HATE myself."

This was the regular way I would chastise myself and I frequently wouldn't leave my house if I had a particularly bad episode that I couldn't cover up.

My friends would always tell me: it's not as bad as you think, I can't see anything, honestly you look fine to me, just a little blotchy that's all, just stick a bit of makeup on it, that will sort it out. Then they would complain if they had just one single little spot come up that interrupted the landscape of their otherwise beautiful skin. In truth they were only trying to be nice. And how could they really understand what was going on in my head and how deeply the state of my skin was affecting me.

I tell you all this. If you have been, or are going through, the "skin "thing there is some hope that it can get better. And I also urge those of you who have normal skin to be kind to those who don't.

I remember not so long ago, travelling to Milan with my eldest daughter for a long weekend. I was fifty-three at the time and having a really bad breakout on my chin. I looked in the mirror in the small bathroom of the hotel room we shared and just burst into tears. I was convinced that I must be the only person in the world to still have acne at the age of fifty-three. But at its root, adult acne is caused by the same things that cause teen acne: excess skin oil and bacteria. I think stress also contributed to my acne and the more I stressed about it, the worse it seemed to get.

Many adults do suffer from adult acne and it really does have a disproportionate mental impact on those who suffer from it. There are many treatments that can help and I did try most of them, but the only one that really worked for me was Isotretinoin capsules (Roaccutane). This treatment is definitely not for everyone and has to be prescribed by a qualified professional as there are various side effects, some serious. I certainly got incredibly dry eyes and dry lips which were difficult to cope with at first. However the treatment made a miraculous difference to me, not just because it stopped my face being like an oil slick 24/7 and my spots completely stopped coming up, but my mental health improved dramatically. If you are really suffering like I did, then getting the right help and being taken seriously for how bad the state of your skin affects your mental health is crucial. So don't suffer behind closed doors. Get some professional help.

I probably spent many thousands of pounds on off the shelf creams and beauty products that did not really work very well. Some seemed to work for a little while but then their effect would wear off. Going to see your GP can be really helpful, but they are quite restricted about what they can prescribe so my advice is, instead of spending vast amounts of money on beauty products, pay to see a recommended dermatologist privately if you can. This goes against my principles in many ways, but actually if you can afford it, I personally think it can really be worth it. It certainly worked for me.

Chapter 2

The curse of anorexia

On the self-loathing theme, my sister has always had a weight problem and she would eat, and probably still does, for comfort. I know that immediately after she has over indulged she feels incredibly guilty. She has done endless diets which have never succeeded and constantly berates herself for not achieving her target weight. I'm not sure mum ever really understood this and would often make very unhelpful comments about my sister's weight, making her feel even more upset. The thing about my sister is, though, that she is beautiful and has amazing skin. She is also very happily married to a wonderful man and was a tremendous support for me when I went through my divorce.

I always thought I would trade being thin with spots (and now wrinkles) for being fat with perfect skin. So many of us are not happy with the way we look and I am not sure there will ever be a solution to this phenomenon. We just have to find a way to give ourselves a break and somehow learn to accept ourselves with all our so called flaws. We all judge people without really truly understanding what they are going through, but now, whenever I feel myself being judgmental I try to remember that I have been judged by many people who don't know the true me. And I try to be tolerant and kind. Kindness is underrated, I feel, in today's chaotic world.

As I got older, I discovered that although my efforts to get my skin looking better failed miserably on a regular basis, the one thing I was really good at, unlike my sister, was controlling my weight. I can honestly say I was an expert.

I can even remember an exact event that gave me the reason to start losing weight.

It was a school performance of some kind. I can't remember what it was for, but part of it involved a gymnastics display. It was 4th year of secondary school so I would have been about 16 – and I actually was quite good at sport – even winning a "sports girl of the year "award earlier that year. But during the display, when I was performing an Arab spring – a sort of cartwheel that ends with a jump, I completely messed it up and the resounding thump that I made landing in the school hall made the whole audience laugh.

I felt utterly embarrassed and just wanted to curl up and die. I really do not know why it affected me so badly. Maybe it was because I always felt people were laughing or talking about me behind my back, perhaps due to my skin, and now I definitely felt it was because I was too fat, and that meant I simply had to lose weight. I may not have been able to sort my skin out, but at least I could be thin. Back then, and to some extent even now, everyone loves and envies thin girls- don't they?

At that time not much was known, or at least there certainly wasn't much said, about anorexia.

Those were the days without mobile phones, the internet or reality TV shows. In fact it still astonishes my children when I remind them that as a teenager I had no mobile phone. I couldn't google an answer to everything. There was no face-book, Instagram, snap chat or twitter. There wasn't even a celebrity culture that so many young children these days seem to aspire to. And there were hardly any magazines showing impossibly perfect women and telling you how you could and should achieve that perfect look.

So I cannot claim to have been unduly influenced by social pressures or the media, unlike the girls, and some boys, of today.

My favourite actress was Audrey Hepburn. She was just beautiful, very romantic and adored by so many. But I guess looking back on it, she happened to have flawless skin and she was also very thin. I think the main reason I decided to control my weight was because I was so good at it, and if I couldn't have the skin that everyone dreamed of, at least I could be thin, which so many of the women I knew also aspired to be.

For me, losing weight became something of an obsession or even an addiction. I began "faking" what I had eaten, almost even convincing myself that I had had breakfast, when in fact I had only had one bite of a piece of dried toast. In reality I had thrown the rest of the toast away, carefully concealing the waste so my mum wouldn't find out. I would make sure there were some crumbs on the plate and even a dirty knife that I had stuck in the jam jar for effect on the plate. I would also make the point to mum that I had had two slices of toast with some lovely jam for breakfast that day, and I had really enjoyed them.

I would invariably say not to worry about lunch or dinner as I was eating with a friend, which I invariably was not. I used to make lists that I wanted to adhere to and would get really upset with myself if I had gone off the rails. If I ate too much I would feel incredibly guilty and loathe myself for it.

I would write lists of dos and don'ts and was convinced that being thin would make me happy.

My mum was worried and even got me a counsellor – who I thought was thinner than me and looked bulimic, so I couldn't take her seriously. My dad just thought the answer was easy - just tell her to eat more! I think it is fair to say that I really did have a distorted image of myself and thought if I could eat less and exercise more I would eventually be a perfect weight.

When my youngest daughter was about fourteen, to my absolute horror she, too, began the miserable toxic journey anorexia spirals you through. Whilst I have recovered (although once you have had an eating disorder I truly don't think you ever are free of it) she continues to suffer, and I blame myself for that on a regular basis. I found her open diary one day whilst tidying her room and it broke my heart. The same self-loathing I had, the same lists of things to eat or not to eat, and how many calories are contained in certain foods and how to secretly achieve weight loss with the aim that being thin will make her happy.

I was anorexic for many years. Spurred on by what I thought were compliments, such as "Ooh, you are looking very slim these days," no doubt meant to be taken as concern not as a compliment. I found pleasure in buying the smallest sizes, that I would then have to take in even further to fit me. I had certain exercise routines that I had to do every day without fail and forced myself to keep them up even if I felt exhausted. I would place a ruler across my stomach at night and be delighted when I could get my hand underneath it whilst it pressed on to each hip bone. If there was any food that tempted me in the flat or house I was living in at the time, then I would throw it in the bin before I gave in to temptation – only to find myself rummaging through the same bin later that night for something to eat.

During studying for my A-levels I joined a drama and dance group where being slim was certainly the norm, and I also lost my virginity. My sister and I were going out with two guys who were best friends at the same time.

I remember being besotted with Gary. He was incredibly popular at the college I was studying at, and the fact he was with me made me feel extra special. He, like most people were unaware of my battle with food, and I had found some make up that, once I had spent an hour applying very carefully, didn't look too bad. I really do not know why he was with me, but perhaps he had guessed I had never had sex before and he got a kick out of being the one to help me lose my virginity.

Soon after we got together he was in a major car accident. One of our friends who was driving was killed. This so called friend used to say, "are you feeling lucky tonight lads," and he would often drive far too fast and probably under the influence. This time he had overtaken going up a hill on a blind bend. There was another car coming directly at him. His car overturned and he had died instantly. The fire and rescue services took several hours to cut Gary out of the wreckage and he was in hospital for months following the accident. Friends and relatives who visited Gary in hospital used to tell him how lucky he was. But actually he didn't feel lucky at all. He felt very angry and he was in a lot of pain. Soon he shunned his hospital visitors, including me, and I was distraught.

There was nothing I could do to change the situation, or to help him. The only thing I could do was to keep controlling my weight so that when he did come out of hospital he would still want to be with me. I did not see him for a long time.

On my 18th birthday, mum and dad said we could have a party at my house and that they would go away for the night to leave us to it. They were pretty relaxed about these kinds of things but also incredibly stupid.

I intended to have a few friends round and had invited Gary to the party even though we hadn't been a couple since his accident. I have literally no idea how a few invited friends became about a random one hundred turning up at the door. Considering we had no mobile phones and no internet I simply have no idea how news of the party got around so quickly. Even people I didn't know turned up, and I let them in. My colourful cousin Sarah came to the party. She had a brief stint as a drummer in a band called the Boomtown Turkeys. I distinctly remember that we put all the furniture out in the garden and she and her band played in the living room. How the police were not called remains a mystery to me.

I learnt only recently that my brother shagged the lead singer of the band that night. She had a bone piercing through her nose and apparently green pubes with "keep off the grass" tattooed on her fanny.

My mum used to ice wedding cakes for a living – in fact she even did Vivian Leigh's wedding cake as I recall. Something for her memoires, I guess. That weekend she had iced a cake for a customer bride-to-be and thought the safest place to put it was in the airing cupboard in the bathroom. Unbelievably, at some point in the evening someone shut themselves in the bathroom and chopped up the cake into little pieces and put them in the bath. I can't quite even remember how mum sorted that one out. We had far too much food which ended up on the floor, and how the place wasn't set on fire with all the smoking I will never know. Drugs were most probably enjoyed, although I have never taken any to this day. I was so thin one large glass of wine was enough for me to lose any sense of what was right or wrong. For a large part of the evening I talked to Gary. We went upstairs and had sex. He had assumed I must have been with someone else over the year we had been apart, and wasn't so gentle with me as he had been on our first and only time. The next morning, apart from the demolished cake, fag butts and food stamped into the carpets, mum also found blood stained sheets in the wash bin.

She never really discussed the whole incident with me and somehow I just carried on as normal even though it had affected me deeply.

CHAPTER 3

The curse of bulimia

After A Levels, I decided, for some unknown reason, I was going to go and do a Sports Science degree. A new degree which sounded lots of fun, and at the same polytechnic as my sister was doing her teaching degree, Nottingham Polytechnic. There are no polytechnics l eft now, they all became full-blown universities in 1992 under the Further and Higher Education Act 1992. Somehow they were looked down upon as a lower form of university – only people who couldn't get into a good Uni went to a Polytechnic and were somehow not as intelligent – which I think was unfair.

I remember thinking I could have even more control of what I ate living away from home. And all the exercise would certainly burn up huge amounts of calories.

The only issue was that when I got there I found out there were only six people on the course – It was such a new course that very few candidates had actually applied to study on it. I could tell after two weeks that this was not going to work. My best sports were team sports and we couldn't even make one side of a basketball team, let alone a hockey team, and hockey was one of my favourite sports. I was still determined to stay put in Nottingham so I rather hurriedly researched other courses on offer at the Polytechnic and found they offered a Dance and Art Degree. This ticked a lot of boxes for me so I decided to apply. I hadn't really thought this all through at all as after a year of Dance you were then supposed to major in Art. I had not thought about the impact of having to drop the dance in a years' time. Undeterred, I bought a sketch pad and spent a weekend frantically drawing. I sketched still lifes and made charcoal drawings of trees and took it to the course director. Amazingly he liked what he saw. He accepted me onto the new course and I switched my degree the following week.

I actually found myself loving the dance, especially as being thin was the norm. So many of the girls on my course restricted what they ate and one of them had learnt how to make herself sick. She shared a book about it with me. I was utterly fascinated and decided that being sick could be the answer to all my issues about weight management.

I found it quite difficult at first, but practice makes perfect and being able to eat what I really craved for was a revelation to me. I could eat what I wanted and just puke it all up after. I became quite an expert at this new kind of weight control. I honed my skills, finding out when the best time to puke was - how long, for example, should you wait after eating before you tried to be sick, how drinking something fizzy would really help, how to make sure my breath didn't smell after each disgusting episode and checking the toilet seat and my clothes extremely carefully after each session to ensure no-one could suspect that I had been sick.

I got so adept at the art of puking on demand that I could even be sick during courses if we went out for a meal. I would try to ensure no-one was in the loo and go out and do the deed as quietly as possible. Carefully washing my hands, spraying breath freshener into my revolting mouth and then re-applying my lipstick so no-one would suspect.

I hated myself even more for my bulimia than I did for my anorexia. At least I had a semblance of control with my anorexia - but I had absolutely no control over this vile disease. Once I had started eating, I couldn't stop – thinking it wouldn't matter. But it did. I remember being given a chocolate gateau one day, probably a birthday "treat". I took it home and stared at it for a very long time. I thought I would just have one slice. No, maybe just half a slice. Surely that would be OK? I thought I would be able to dance off the calories or run around the block a few times. I took a bite. The sweet, sugary, delicious chocolate cake melting in my mouth was incredible, especially as I had been denying myself chocolate for so long. But even as I ate it I started thinking, could I eat a whole slice and get away with it? Thinking about eating a slice and getting away with it soon turned to planning how it might be possible to eat more than one slice and puke it up. Once I had eaten one slice there seemed little point in stopping there so I began devouring slice after slice, with tears streaming down my face as I finished the last one. Then I ran to the fridge and started drinking diet coke to enable the horrendous process of vomiting up as much of my indulgence as possible. Fingers down the back of my throat.

Desperately hoping I could bring most of it up. Temporary relief as the cake spewed out into the toilet bowl. Looking at my red swollen eyes in the mirror and feeling like the most disgusting person that ever lived.

Not only would I make myself vomit, I also abused laxatives. I would often take several tablets at a time in the hope I could shit away the excess calories. This had mixed results and was clearly really bad for me, too.

My relationship with bulimia lasted for many years and probably never stopped until I was pregnant with my first child. It truly is the most revolting mental health problem. At the time I did not really understand the long term health issues. And even if I did, I am not sure I could have stopped myself from purging. Bulimia can lead to electrolyte imbalances which affect the heart rate and the function of other major organs, including the kidneys. Bulimics are at risk of heart failure, kidney failure and even death, and sadly eating disorders kill more people than any other mental illness in the UK. Sufferers are more likely to commit suicide, self-harm in other ways or experience organ failure. Half of women will recover from bulimia within ten years of their diagnosis, but an estimated 30% of these women will relapse. Clearly I am very lucky that somehow I was able to recover from this self-destructive illness.

During my year at Nottingham, I fell in love with contemporary dancing. It was a real shame that I wasn't that good at it. I wish I could say the same about art, as I found the art course incredibly disappointing. As it happens, I actually do have a very artistic family – my mum is a watercolour artist, and my eldest daughter is also an amazing painter. There are also many musicians and dancers in my family. So perhaps I should have enjoyed the art course more.

It turned out that I was surprisingly very good at drawing and painting almost photographic looking pictures – but I think that they lacked soul and originality. And my teachers, in any case, were into very modern unorthodox art.

So, for my end of term appraisal I decided to try and see what would happen if I just put some old pieces of wood together, chuck on some paint, glue on a bit of whatever I could find in the kitchen and pretend it was an expression of my inner feelings meant to portray the twisted agony of dealing with fitting in – or some such bollocks.

I presented my masterpiece to my tutor, ready for some deserved criticism, but to my surprise he thought it was fantastic. He praised me for thinking so intensely about such a personal topic. I think I even got an A which was utter madness. I never owned up.

As I mentioned earlier, after the first year you were required to drop dance and just study art. I knew that there was no way that I could do that and I just had to find another place to continue dance and hopefully a degree.

I auditioned for the Laban School of Movement and Dance - a highly prestigious University, part of University of Goldsmiths in London. I choreographed a dance to some panpipe music and danced in front of a judging panel. I was a nervous wreck and unsure as to what the panel would think of this skinny, awkward, but flexible dancer. Amazingly however, I actually got in. I was utterly overwhelmed and truly believed a new start could be everything I had ever dreamed of. Maybe I could sort my mental and physical health out.

But my dreams, however, were soon to be crushed. Two weeks before the start of the degree I was told by my County Council in Somerset that they would not fund it. Although the degree was a BA (Hons) in Dance Theatre, due to the element of dance, they were not obliged to fund it. In those days UCAS didn't exist as it does now.

My parents were not well off and couldn't afford to fund me and so there was no way I could go.

Utterly devastated I thought, what the fuck next?

Chapter 4

Off to London

Bizarrely to keep fit I had taken a course in the summer to become an aerobics teacher – just something I thought might be useful as it was all the rage at the time. The image of Jane Fonda wearing leotard and leg warmers has become really iconic. And the saying "feel the burn" was coined at that time.

I am certain the course I took was not accredited in any way, shape or form, and certainly didn't give me a qualification to teach, but, nevertheless I came up with a slightly bonkers idea.

I would go to London and hold my own aerobics classes. I would take my rather dodgy "qualification" certificate with me and make a living out of teaching keep fit. I still look back on this crazy decision and think, 'how on earth did I actually do this?'.

I got on an overnight coach from Taunton to London Victoria, with no idea where I was going to live, no friends in London, no job and just a little cash my mum had given me. Why mum and dad never tried to talk me out of it I will never know.

Bearing in mind that I had no mobile phone either, how stupid was I? A skinny 19 year old girl with a large case, landing in London on a grey morning in September, utterly exhausted after virtually no sleep, and without a clue.

I followed signs in the station so that I could put my case in storage and then remember making my way to Covent Garden, because even then that was considered to be "trendy". My first task was to find somewhere to live fast, and so I picked up some kind of magazine which had various ads for bed-sits to rent in the back pages. I knew I needed somewhere to live that day, and my plan was to find a small room to rent. I had to use a public phone box to make lots of calls and was soon running out of coins. Every bedsit that I thought might suit me and in the right price bracket seemed to have already been taken. I was getting very worried. I thought I might have to give this ridiculous idea up and go back home or end up sleeping rough on the streets. However, literally the last one on the list was an advert for a small bedsit to rent in a house opposite Earls Court Station and it was still available. The landlord answered my call within a couple of rings and said he was taking viewings from about lunchtime. I was hugely relieved and made my way there immediately, only to join a relatively long queue of young people who were also there to view the "small" bedsit.

Small, was a bit of an exaggeration. It was miniscule. It was the size of a single bed in fact. The single bed which filled the small red carpeted floor, folded away to allow space for you to enter the room. It had a teeny corner sink and an equally tiny fridge up on the wall. It was very dark and there was a strange smell about the house. Either it was the Chinese man who rented the flat in the basement below, and continually had something cooking on his stove, or perhaps it was the mysterious Italian man on the first floor who definitely was smoking something illegal. It could have just been blocked drains, I guess.

There was a shared bathroom on the first floor, which later I discovered always seemed to be permanently occupied by the Italian. One day, when he had been in the toilet for what seemed like hours, I was so desperate for a shit I literally had to poo in a saucepan in my room. I then had to wait another hour before I could dispose of it. Naturally I had to throw that pan away later.

There also seemed to be a fair amount of mildew and slightly peeling magnolia paint up the stair case.

Funny really how no-one really wanted it – but I wasn't put off at all. I only needed a small bed and definitely only needed a small fridge all things considered. I gave the landlord a cash deposit there and then, with a plan to sign on at the nearest job centre the following Monday. I didn't tell the landlord I would be on benefits, which was probably a good thing as I am sure he would not have let the room to me if he knew. He said that I could move in later that day after I signed all the necessary paperwork. I can't really understand how happy I was initially, to have this tiny space to call my own. My next task was to find somewhere to keep fit, and potentially work out how I was going to start holding some of my own aerobics classes. There was so much for me to think about but I knew there was somewhere I did want to go first.

I had read about a relatively new dance place, called The Pineapple Dance Studio, that had opened in Convent Garden a couple of years before I landed in London. It is still extremely successful to this day, and now has around twelve dance studios, and hosts over two-hundred dance classes a week.

I made my way there not knowing exactly what I really wanted to do. It was a membership only club, although you could pay individually for classes. The problem for me was that I did not have the money to join. Undeterred by this obvious issue I walked straight in without looking at anyone on reception and managed to attend many classes without paying anything. Incredibly, and much to my disgust looking back on it now, I did get away with this approach for some time after. I attended lots of different classes, but a contemporary class run by a small Chinese male dancer was my favourite.

There was a small coffee bar and one back wall where various information and the occasional jobs were posted. The first day I went to Pineapple I saw an advert posted on the wall for an aerobics teacher in a sports centre in Camden. They needed someone for two evenings a week to teach a beginners and then an advanced class. In today's world where everyone needs to have a DBS Check and proof of qualifications, getting a job teaching in this manor would have been very difficult for someone like me. But back then things were less regulated and there were less checks on everything we did. I simply called up the manager and told him I was qualified and ready to take the classes and he asked me to come and meet him. So I met him later that day and incredibly he gave me the job straight away.

It's funny looking back on it how different fitness classes were in those days. I know that I went back home on the coach and collected my car that week which was a mustard coloured Austin Maestro, and it was as awful as it sounds (I definitely made some very poor choices when it came to cars). I picked up my huge heavy ghetto blaster, a bunch of tapes and an old record player. I made my own tapes up for my classes, recording the tracks for "warm ups," "runs," "legs and bums," "stomachs" and "stretch and cool down". I found a great record shop in Brixton and bought 12" singles to use for each section. I still have those records today.

There were no microphones back then so you had to shout whilst you tried to demonstrate and do the classes. I loved it at the time and my classes became very popular. Every self-respecting woman would have a lycra leotard and leg warmers and wanted a bit of Jane Fonda, and to feel the burn. I once had over a hundred people in the class which probably sounds ridiculous, but it was true. Unfortunately after a while it did take a toll on my voice. I completely lost it at one point and I was told strictly not to speak for at least 2 weeks for fear of permanent vocal damage. That was tough. It's quite hard running an exercise class from the front without being able to speak.

Alongside the small income I received from doing these classes, I rented a studio out at Pineapple. It cost me £8 per hour to rent the studio, which seemed quite a lot to me, but one day I had a whole coach load of Japanese tourists come in to Pineapple to try out a Jane Fonda style class in the studio which was becoming famous.

I couldn't believe my luck. I took £3 per tourist and had thirty-five in my class. The only problem for me was my studio was so tiny, probably ten would have been a good size class and if all the tourists attempted a star jump at the same time they would have knocked each other down. Thankfully the Japanese are quite small as a rule, and I quickly adapted my class to suit the space and just about got away with it.

I also found work in a fitness and dance studio in Clapham called The Other Side of the Track, and in the exclusive Chelsea Dance Studios. I remember a young Martin Clunes, best known now for portraying Martin Ellingham in the ITV drama series, Doc Martin, coming to one of my aerobics classes there, and I think I nearly killed him. Sorry Martin! Unsurprisingly, he never came back.

To top up all of my earnings I also got a job as a waitress in a restaurant in Brixton. I was soon earning enough to move from my miniscule bedsit to a small flat in Anerley, near Crystal Palace. Ainsley Harriot was the chef for the restaurant there just before he got famous. He was delightful. Warm and funny, and a joy to work with. I remember at that time he was also in a band called Calypso Twins – and a few of my friends and I would watch them perform at the Comedy Club on Lavender Hill. I first saw Julian Clary and Fanny the Wonder Dog perform there, although I can't recall the dog doing anything in particular. A couple of years ago I got back in touch with Ainsley via his agent and he actually rang me back and left a lovely voicemail message saying it would be great to catch up. Sadly he didn't leave a contact number and I just felt it might be stalking if I tried to get in touch again. Who knows, maybe if this book gets published I might send him a copy and maybe I will get to say hello again.

In April 1981, Brixton like many parts of UK, was affected by a recession. There were a lot of serious social and economic problems, but the Afro Caribbean community had particularly high unemployment, poor housing and a high crime rate. There had been growing unease between police and the local people. A group of young black residents died in a fire that was suspected to be a racially motivated arson.

Marching and protests followed and tensions erupted following an incident where a young boy died after a stabbing. It was claimed that this was a result of police brutality.

I had arrived at the restaurant to do my shift at around 4:30pm on the Saturday, 11th April 1981. I remember sensing something was wrong and listening to the local radio filling us in on what was happening. The restaurant was just off Acre Lane, one of the many areas where shops were later looted. We soon knew a riot was in progress, and could hear loud screams and shouts, bottles and bricks being thrown and angry marching youths.

We locked the door. Only one couple had turned up for their early dinner reservation, the rest had obviously heard the news about what was going on and had wisely decided not to go out in the Brixton area that night.

But during the evening the door was kicked open and 10 youths wearing black balaclavas rushed in, demanding money. One held a large knife up to my face and asked me to empty the till. There really wasn't much money in the till so he took the couple's cards and jewellery from them. There was hugely expensive wine, whiskeys and other spirits behind the bar but surprisingly they just asked for bottles of Perrier. I think they, too, seemed rather scared. And then they ran off.

I am not sure how we secured the door but we spent the rest of the night upstairs looking out of the window at the rioters. The couple who had their cards stolen stayed with us and sheltered in the restaurant.

There was a tyre shop opposite us and I remember the large front window being smashed and several cars parking up outside and taking whatever sets of tyres they wanted.

Later that evening some vans also parked up opposite the restaurant opening their doors and revealing various household appliances which they offered out to people – I guess the word had spread. There was a lot of looting that night. It was dubbed "Bloody Saturday" by the Times although no-one died. I think there were about 300 injuries to police, 50 to members of the public and over 100 vehicles burned. Over 5000, people were involved.

By this time I had left the Austin Metro I had been driving ashamedly around in, somewhere on Chelsea Embankment and bought a delightful frog-green fiat for £300 – dubbed the Snot Mobile by my friends. A kid had once shot at me with an air rifle, but the screen hadn't broken – it just had a cracked spider's web look about it. It also didn't have a hand brake that worked. I had to park it in gear, especially if on a hill.

Oh how I would have loved that car to be set on fire at the time of the riots - the 2 cars parked either side of it on the first night of the riots had been totally burned out but mine had somehow been left alone. Later, in an attempt to get my car stolen so I could claim on the insurance, I even tried leaving the keys in the ignition for 2 weeks over Christmas. I returned in the new year only to find it was still there.

There was still trouble on the Sunday of that weekend and there were many police cordons set up. I tried to drive home but could see I needed to find another route. I stopped the car whilst considering my options – engine still running. To my horror a policeman tapped on the passenger window and asked, 'where are you trying to go?'. He then proceeded to hop in next to me to give me some support. He said – "turn off the engine love" – and to be helpful, he pulled up the hand brake – which of course was not attached – to reveal a hole in the car floor (quite a handy hole if you wanted to throw away the odd banana skin or two whilst driving). Quickly thinking, I remarked, "Ooh look what you've done officer!" Not sure he was convinced he'd done it, but he rather kindly suggested I had it fixed or face a three point fixed penalty and a fine. Luckily I got away with that one.

I previously said I had made a few duff car choices. I think buying second hand cars when you were young was easy in the 1980s, as the insurance really didn't cost much compared to the price of the car, and I just don't remember there being so many checks.

The Maestro had had a lot of gear problems and at one point I simply could not get it in to reverse. Parking was a particular nightmare as I would have to leave it in neutral, get out and push it back to try and manoeuvre it into a space – which, as a skinny young woman, was not that easy. I would often ask for the assistance of a helpful passer-by, if they looked friendly.

One day after a class at the Chelsea Dance Studios I made a real effort with the gear stick and was delighted when I finally got it into reverse. My joy was soon over though, when I realized it was completely stuck in reverse. The car was worth very little anyway, and so I just left it there on Chelsea Embankment. To this day I don't know what happened to it.

Other cars I had dubious relationships with included a Renault 4 which had no heating and was freezing during the winter snow. It also had no grip and I remember sliding all the way down Crystal Palace Hill narrowly missing many pedestrians and other cars, literally by millimetres. I sold it to a nice guy shortly afterwards and as he drove away the exhaust dropped off. He turned the car around and came back towards me. I was convinced he was going to go mad at me - but instead he just asked for some rope to tie it back on again. He had only bought the car for parts, so I didn't need to worry.

I once had a blue Marina which I quite liked at the time as it was nice and warm. But this car often needed a bump start. Once I had parked it on the top floor of a multistorey car park in Croydon and when I went to drive home late one evening, about 11pm, I could not get it to start. I had a bright idea. I would put the car in first gear, push it down the exit ramp and jump in just as it started up. I know this sounds insane, but I really did do this. The carpark floor was on a slight slope so I did manage to get it going, only then to realize it was too late to jump in as it built up a little speed, and crashed into the wall of the exit ramp.

Having no idea what to do next I went down to the ground floor to make a call. Some bloke was in the phone box and when he had finished his call he got out and noticed I was a little distressed. Amazingly he said he had a tow rope in his boot and he would help me out. He drove to the top of the carpark, managed to pull my car out of the wall and then helped me bump start it. I just don't know how I got away with this kind of thing. I did a lot of slightly risky things back then, but perhaps we all did. With no mobiles, or instant access to the internet maybe we just weren't aware of the dangers we put ourselves in. I guess this total stranger could have taken advantage of me, but I honestly didn't feel scared despite it being nearly midnight and nobody else was around. I did, and still do, always tend to think the best of people.

I once had a cute white mini-metro. One day I was driving on the M25 when it started to overheat. I genuinely thought it was on fire and pulled over on the hard shoulder and called the fire brigade. Soon after I heard the sirens and a huge fire engine pulled up behind me and 12 burly firemen got out. Wonderful guys.

It didn't take them long to discover it wasn't on fire but that the fan belt had broken. Again, I seem to have been lucky with getting help. One particularly muscly fireman asked if I would be happy to take my tights off - to make a temporary fan belt with, of course. I did my best to remove my tights – thank god I was wearing knickers that day - and duly passed them over.

I have no idea how he got the car going with this temporary fix, but he offered to help me get a new fan belt fitted as he knew of a garage nearby that we could get one from. I can't quite remember what happened next, but he came with me to the garage and helped to fit the new belt which is apparently a sod to do on a mini metro. There was an accident and he cut his arm really badly. He had to go to hospital and have 38 stiches. I felt so guilty – not only because he hurt himself but because I never did get back in touch to thank him.

I have had some lovely cars since working in the pharmaceutical industry – where I still enjoy a really rewarding career. Most of my troubles have been to do with getting speeding or parking tickets since having company cars.

My first company car was a bright red Ford Sierra and I thought it was utterly amazing. I drove it home with the music on full blast, going idiotically fast on the M20, and promptly got pulled over. I was really lucky not to be banned, but when I burst in to tears in front of the officers and told them it was my first day of work, they let me off with a fine and three points. It wasn't the last time crying my heart out in front of two policemen got me out of trouble.

One time, I put washer fluid in to the place oil is meant to go … I really should learn some more about cars …

I did all kinds of jobs in London. After being knackered and not earning enough trying to juggle running my own aerobic classes, and topping up with waitressing work, I got a job running the small café bar and doing classes at a fitness studio in Croydon. I turned my hand to selling paintings. I became a manager at an upper-class burger restaurant in Chiswick. I worked in a bank. I worked in bars.

I even sold computer training courses, which was hilarious considering I had never even owned a computer or even switched one on. This was tele sales and I found myself surprisingly good at it.

Our sales offices were in Clerkenwell Road. It was a large space with about twenty of us working in it. We were given a geographical area and the equivalent of a phone directory to cold call businesses. My area was Essex and Hertfordshire. We all smoked as we worked in the office. I didn't particularly even like smoking, but found I quite enjoyed the taste and look of More Menthols. To keep my breath fresher I would first put a polo mint in my mouth and then smoke this long dark brown slim cigarette. We must have all stank by the end of the day and I just cannot quite understand how we all put up with each other puffing away all day. The habit of sucking polos whilst smoking, combined with the bulimia no doubt contributed significantly to the state of my teeth which eventually, in a roundabout way, lead to the birth of my first daughter.

I became quite good at cold calling random companies and selling them our training courses: Word for Windows,

Excel, SMART and so forth. This was despite the fact that I had no idea what these things were. There was a large board on the front wall of the office with a table and all our names listed. Whenever we got a sale we would march up to the board and cross off the total value of the courses we had sold in cash. There was a line drawn to the right hand side of the board and this represented the target you aimed to hit each month. If you sold enough courses you would then start earning commission. Everyone in the office would applaud when you walked up to put a sale on the board, but be secretly jealous when you got a sale that took you past the target line.

I always seemed to just about get to the commission line at the very last minute – which pissed a lot of others off but made me laugh. I had made a great contact with a manager from Thurrock Borough Council and he never failed to help me out. He always faxed me across a booking if I needed it right at the last minute. His name was John, and he sounded so sexy on the phone.

As he had given me so much business I was allowed to meet him and take him to lunch. We had been flirting quite a lot on the phone and I had built up a picture of him in my mind. I was convinced he was young, perhaps late 30s. Tall with dark hair and a boyish smile.

I was so excited to be meeting him finally and had put on a slightly too short skirt with a slightly too low blouse for work. I got myself very worked up and had already thought about what we might do on a second date.

However, we never did have that second date. When he came in to the restaurant I was totally shocked. He was probably in his late 50s, overweight, balding on top with large sideburns and glasses. He also had a pronounced limp, had a walking stick and one shoe that was built up to try to even out the limp.

I was utterly deflated and inside felt incredibly stupid. What on earth had I been thinking, it couldn't have been worse. Although, of course, in reality it could have been worse; and he was actually very nice, and we were in a safe environment. I learnt a lot from this situation which helped me prepare for many of the blind dates I was to have later on in my life.

I lived in many different bedsits during my first time in London. The Earls Court bedsit, although convenient, was never going to be anywhere I could stay too long. I lived in Crystal Palace, Anerley, Brixton, Forest Hill, Nunhead, and later even in Hounslow.

Life was so busy, but in many ways lonely as moving around and changing jobs all the time meant that I was finding it difficult to make lasting friendships. It also wasn't good for my health. Living on your own when you have an eating disorder is probably the worst thing you can do. Especially when you have told no-one of your condition and secretly hate yourself for it every day.

Something one day made me realize I had to go back to Somerset where I grew up and re-think where and what I was going to do. I truly believed I would be coming back to London once I had finally got my shit together. I resigned from all my various jobs and paid my last rent. I packed up my car and drove home wondering if everything I had been doing had been a complete waste of time. Mum and Dad were, in truth, really supportive and welcomed me back with open arms. I didn't know how I would find living back with my parents, but it wasn't as bad as I thought it would be. I was still only 21 and I was sure I could get a job back in London at some point.

Meanwhile a new shop was opening in the nearby town of Taunton. It was a Body Shop – not the car kind, but the skincare kind. Dame Anita Roddick founded the Body Shop in 1976 and it became, and still is, amazingly successful.

Somehow I got a job as an assistant manager there, and later, the manager. The shop was run by two wealthy franchisees. They said all the right things publicly in line with the Body Shop ethos, but behind closed doors they were anything but ethical.

I met Anita Roddick when the shop opened and she was lovely but utterly bonkers. She was a real activist. She formed an alliance with Greenpeace and the whole concept of the Body Shop appealed to me greatly. She was anti-capitalist and against globalization. Although later she was happy to be known as a capitalist with a conscience. The Body Shop supported fair trade with communities that supposedly needed it the most and was absolutely totally against testing of any cosmetics on animals.

I do remember going up on a coach to London with a group of employees and storming the Brazilian Embassy to protest about their record in animal cruelty.

There was however later a lot of controversy surrounding all the claims Anita Roddick had made, and the business practices of the Body Shop. Anita herself died of a heart attack, aged 62, on the 10th of September 2007 – (ironically my birthday). She had had hepatitis C for 30 years.

I loved my work initially. It was really exciting to be part of a new shop opening and I worked really hard. When I became acting manager I ended up with a large number of staff to look after; I think around 14 at one point. My role included ensuring the day to day running of the shop went smoothly, organizing staff rotas, banking the takings at the end of each day, doing staff training and general managerial duties. But things went sour when the girl who had hoped to be promoted to manager instead of me, plotted her revenge.

Thinking back on working at the shop, I do remember once selling Charles Dance a bottle of banana conditioner, and this in turn reminded me of all the brief encounters I have had with various celebrities over the years.

It is also slightly worrying that most of them are dead now.

I met Eric Morecambe and have a picture of me sitting on his knee when I was about twelve. I said hello to Phil Lynott from Thin Lizzy at a nightclub in Soho. I met

Keith Chegwin during Saturday Swap Shop. Probably something to do with my age ...

Anyway, long story short involving my hair turning bright orange after trying out a "natural" hair dye, funds being taken from the charity box and hurricane force winds leading to me closing the shop five minutes early one day, I ended up getting unfairly and instantly dismissed. And so closed that chapter.

Time to find a new career – one which I have stayed with all my life now.

One of my friends had come in to the body shop one day and said she was working in the pharmaceutical industry and I should try it. Bearing in mind I didn't have a degree, and not even an A Level in science, I thought she was mad at the time. But after I had been sacked form the Body Shop I thought, what did I have to lose?

Through my friend's network I got an interview with Bayer Pharmaceuticals and with the support of this amazing friend I unbelievably got my first job in Pharma.

Pharmaceutical Sales Representative - is the kind of secret but brilliant job I would recommend to anyone. So many Pharma Reps I have known over the years complain about the erratic hours, long drives, useless computer system, crap bonus scheme, annoying boss, difficult customers, really don't know how lucky they are. We get paid more than the average doctor, we get a company car, (nice car) a company pension, private health – the list is endless. Yes its stressful, and yes, you have to do loads of admin and lots of rather silly sales training courses and you have to be away from home a bit. But if you are good at it and believe in what you are selling, then it's an incredibly rewarding, well-paid job.

If you have never watched Love and other Drugs, a 2010 film starring Jake Gyllenhaal as a handsome Pharmaceutical Sales Rep, I would highly recommend it. Equally hilarious and sad, it gives a rather unflattering glimpse into my world, which I hope has changed somewhat since then.

Getting the job with Bayer enabled me to return to London. At last, I thought, I could start afresh in the City I loved and hated in equal measures.

This time I got a bedsit in Hounslow. It was so much nicer than my very first bedsit had been, and I had a swanky new company car to drive around in.

It was during my first job in pharma that I met my eldest daughter's father. I shall return to him later.

With more money to spend I also began trying out various beauty treatments in the hope that I would be more attractive and happier in my own skin.

Chapter 5

Beauty is supposed to be in the eye of the beholder…

Where do I start with the many treatments I have inflicted upon myself in the pursuit of a more attractive face and body? Not just my skin either. I have had quite a few disasters with my rather lacklustre, short, and boring, thinning hair. I remember my dad saying a woman's hair was her crowning glory. What a load of complete bollocks when you have hair like mine.

So! Deep breath, as there are quite a few.

The first major body transformation I went for was probably the biggest one I have subjected myself to, and I am still not ready to give them up just yet 20 years ago, and this was after my third child was born, I decided to have a boob job. I hadn't been thinking about it for long and certainly hadn't done very much research. I didn't even know anyone back then who had had implants or plastic surgery of any kind but I seem to recall reading an advert for a free consultation where you could get advice and supposedly an unbiased opinion from a caring practitioner about what treatments you could have. It came with a promise that their treatments would be carried out by experts in the field of cosmetic surgery and they would be easily affordable. They offered a simple payment plan to entice you to sign up for surgery that would enhance your natural beauty, and change your life for the better.

I used to, and still do, to a certain extent, look at myself in the mirror and see someone who is too fat, too wrinkly, too spotty, too hairy, too ugly, and whose feet are too big, hair is too thin, teeth not white enough, and so forth. I am also born with a hugely annoying tendency to seek perfection, so I couldn't resist the opportunity to go and discuss my flaws and their possible fixes with someone who could understand my craving to look beautiful.

I went in for my free consultation at a local hotel where two rooms had been hired out by the Cosmetic Surgery Company. As I sat in the waiting room with several other women, who all looked really anxious, I wondered what they were thinking about having done. None of them looked like they needed anything doing if you asked me. And yet here we all were, flicking through glossy magazines showing 'before and after' pictures. Articles by women who said having their nose job or their boob job was the best thing they had ever done and praising the skills and care of the surgeon who had performed the operations. I had practically decided already that I would go through with whatever was suggested to me in that consultation.

My turn came and I was called in to the consulting room to be greeted by a very beautiful, amazingly-proportioned young woman who smiled an impossibly perfect smile, and I sat down to discuss how I could be, let's face it, a little more like her. She was kind and listened to my self-loathing tales of how nothing seemed to fit me anymore. How I had lost any resemblance of a decent figure following my third child and my boobs had disappeared completely. Added to that I just couldn't get rid of an annoying tummy bulge, despite all the hundreds of sit ups I was doing on a daily basis, and the healthy diet I was eating.

After just 30 minutes I had signed up for a boob job and she managed to persuade me to go for liposuction on my stomach. The beautiful lady kindly pointed out, whilst I was under general anaesthetic, I may as well have the liposuction, too, as it would be cheaper doing both at the same time instead of separately, considering I was already in theatre. I was very happy with this and the fact that I could pay in instalments.

I was booked in for surgery following a consultation with the doctor who was going to be my surgeon a couple of weeks later. Before I went in to meet my surgeon, I met a couple of ladies in the waiting room who were there for their post-op consultation. They had huge boobs that sat on their chest like giant footballs, and they said I should go really big as they had regretted not having the next size up! I knew I didn't want it to look like a couple of blancmanges had been superglued to my ribcage, so I thought best stick to my plans re getting a nice 34D.

I'm not sure what was worse: revealing my flat chest so that my pathetic looking tits could be poked and prodded and receiving comments like, "I can understand why you've decided to have this operation" and, "how big do you want to go," or having to roll down my trousers and unflattering big knickers to the sound of "mmmmmmm" and "I see what you mean".

Anyway, the doctor was reassuring, professional and gave me the facts and risks involved. I chose to ignore the risks and focused solely on what my new body could look like. I convinced myself that there was nothing wrong with just trying to make yourself look better, and anyway loads of people were having plastic surgery these days.

My ex-husband was with me and supported my decision for surgery. I don't know why he didn't try to talk me out of it but he didn't. Perhaps he knew that I had already made my mind up and he would not have been able to stop me going through with it anyway.

I remember feeling really excited and scared at the same time on the day of the surgery. I counted backwards whilst lying on the trolley as the cold anaesthetic was delivered into my veins and I thought – "it's too late now…"

I woke up feeling utterly battered and bruised all over, and my first thoughts, strangely, weren't about how the operation had gone but just real relief that I was alive. I've had a fear of dying all my life which has actually turned into outright anger now. I used to have nightmares about it but now I seem to be able to change the subject in my head. Why do we have to die, for fuck's sake? As if getting old wasn't bad enough, we all have to die which kind of makes everything we do completely pointless. I've heard there's a place in South London where you can be cryogenically frozen when you die, in the hope that at some point in the future you can be thawed out when technology advances enough to bring you back to life. The thing is, what's the point of being brought back to life in an old person's body? I think maybe I should just freeze my brain, like Walt Disney has done, which is what really makes up my identity and then when technology is advanced enough, bring me back to life and grow a new healthy, perfect body around me. This could be repeated on an ongoing basis. Eventually however, the earth is going to be swallowed up by the sun and we will all end up in a giant black hole, so I guess our existence will have been totally pointless anyway.

I digress. Back to the boob job and liposuction.

I was trussed up in various bandages and ultra-tight fat pants which were designed to keep the swelling under control and improve the healing. I had to wear these for 2 weeks all day and night long.

I was told to try to massage my boobs to keep down the risk of scarring and monitor them regularly before my planned post-operative check-up. I was driven home the same day feeling woozy, in a lot of pain and every corner that the car turned or minor bump we went over absolutely killed me. But to this day I do not regret what I had done, and even whilst I went through pretty agonizing recovery over the weeks following, I absolutely love having bigger boobs. I still do. And I am going to get them redone at some point. As I write this my boobs are twenty years old and still going strong. I have now heard that whilst you are having no problems with your implants and they are still looking and feeling good, then you don't need to get then replaced. Whilst this advice is really welcome, I am so scared that my boobs will burst if I have a mammogram, that I have never had one. My logic tells me I should be screened like all women, especially as I am over fifty-five, but I simply do not want them to burst. I tell myself that after my wedding I will pay for a private MRI scan and that should be able to spot if anything is wrong. I know this is stupid logic but I simply cannot help the way I feel. I do check myself for lumps though and consider myself low risk because I don't smoke, am not obese and no one in my family has ever had breast cancer. I really am such an idiot.

Whilst I loved my new boobs, and the liposuction clearly got rid of my tummy bulge, I have always regretted having that done. This is because when I bend over my stomach looks like a deflated balloon and still to this day I am extremely self-conscious about it. I might be a size ten, but I hate wearing bikinis and nearly always wear stomach supporting swimsuits. My partner constantly tells me that there's absolutely nothing wrong with my stomach and that I look great in bikinis. But as for most of us women with these types of hang-ups, it's how we perceive ourselves to be that drives our self-loathing, no matter what others tell us.

Some years after my boob and tummy job I went in for my next bout of cosmetic surgery – which was driven by an accident in the bath, an idea driven by the media that my fanny wasn't pretty, and a comment my mum made to me when I asked her opinion.

The bath incident was not funny at all.

I realize now that fanny's come in all shapes and sizes (as do cocks of course) And we really should love our own fanny whatever its appearance. And the idea that something is wrong if your fanny is not completely perfect if it doesn't look like a smooth hairless peach is, well quite frankly, ridiculous.

Well, I think possibly because I am quite thin, or just because it was the way I was born, my inner flaps (labia minora) protruded out from my outer flaps (labia majora). About the time that the cosmetic surgery industry really started to take off there was a growing trend to have a "designer vagina" and due to my lack of self-confidence I thought this could potentially fix yet another problem I didn't really have.

I used to have a rather strange landing strip of pubic hair, which I thought might help to cover up the protruding labia minora and one day whilst in the bath I decided it needed a bit of a trim. I lay back and took a little snip off my hair – only to realize that I had accidently also snipped a bit of my inner flap off. It was very, very painful at the time and the bath literally turned a deep shade of blood-red. That rather unfortunate incident made up my mind for me – I definitely needed to have fanny surgery.

I remember asking my mum, which was stupid really as she had only ever seen her own bits, if mine was normal. And her answer was that she didn't think inner flaps usually hung down like the way I described to her, and well, hers certainly didn't, anyway. I wish I had been able to look at something like Jamie McCartney's The Great Wall of Vagina. Maybe then I would have been happy with my own fanny. On May 6th 2011 he was to unveil a nine-metre wall sculpture composed entirely of vulvas. Four hundred fannies. Each the result of a different woman visiting his studio and basically spreading her legs so he could make a cast of it.

This piece of work followed a big trend in women having labiaplasties or designer vaginas, without proper knowledge. I had fallen into the trap of believing my fanny was not in some way attractive and different to everyone else's. All fannies are different in the same way all cocks are. I just wish I hadn't felt my fanny had to be perfectly nice and neat without anything sticking out.

After the bath incident and a bit of time for healing I booked in to have my vagina designed. Again my ex-husband supported my decision - or in any case didn't try to persuade me not to go through with it. This procedure was done in a day under general anaesthetic and I was left with stitches which would supposedly dissolve within a couple of weeks. They did not. So I ended up rather painfully snipping them with a pair of small nail scissors and pulling them out with my tweezers. Do I regret having this surgery, probably. Not only because of the waste of money, but also because of the pain; and I now believe it was a total waste of time, too. I guess my fanny is a bit "tidier" than it was but in no way is it any more attractive.

It's totally clear to me that the more I tried to achieve perfection, the more imperfect I perceived myself to be. I claim to be a feminist and yet I do not seem to act on a personal level in a way that a feminist ought to.

Definition of a feminist-

"Advocating social, political, legal and economic rights for women, equal to those of men.'

I don't see too many men putting themselves through what I did, and still do to a certain extent, in order to satisfy a never ending need to look "what they perceive to be more attractive, more acceptable, more like the ideal." I do appreciate, however, that there are a lot more young men with eating disorders and other anxiety issues than perhaps there was when I was younger.

Due to the nature of my job in the pharmaceutical industry I also crossed paths with those working in the cosmeceutical industry. Cosmeceuticals are products which combine the effects of both cosmetics and pharmaceuticals. One of my friends Claire, was a breast implant sales rep.

She had a lot of friends who also worked in that industry. They sold everything from breast implants to Botox, and all sorts of various forms of fillers. They sold machines to resurface your skin or permanently remove unwanted hair. I was quite excited about the prospect of getting some highly discounted beauty treatments.

Very often those who worked in the industry needed "models" to showcase their products, and of course I volunteered for everything. After all it wasn't just discounted, it was free. All I had to agree to do was I to allow my photo to be used for promotion. This was literally a dream come true for me. I gave my number out to all her friends who might need a model to try some product or procedure on. I was convinced that all the products and procedures must be safe, and assumed they had all been clinically proven. Each time I went to try something I had to read all the small print but in truth I would just sign at the bottom, pretty much ignoring all the possible side effects.

I was a "model" for all sorts of fillers, facial resurfacing products and procedures such as chemical peels and lasering. I bruise quite easily so often I would have to go to work for a couple of weeks following a procedure with a swollen face and black eyes. I didn't want to admit what I was having done, so I would make a stupid excuse up like I had had a dental extraction that had gone wrong, or I would say that I had fallen over drunk. Let's face it, they all knew my love of Sav Blanc. Anything rather than admit I was being a stupid narcissistic, vain idiot trying to make a silk purse out of a sow's ear as the saying goes. I can't believe it but as I am writing this I have an appointment booked to potentially have more fillers in my cheeks. I should be certified.

One of the procedures came back to haunt me a couple of years after I had it done, and it continues to be an ongoing problem.

I was offered an opportunity to be a hand model for a new procedure which would make my aging hands look more youthful. Basically, this involved having a special type of filler injected into the back of my hands. This was supposed to make my hands look less veiny, and encourage the growth of collagen around where the injections had been, in order to smooth out the surface of the back of the hand. I had this procedure done at the Royal College of Medicine in London by a top International cosmetic surgeon, and it was watched by quite a large audience. This novel treatment would have cost hundreds, if not thousands of pounds and the fact I was having this done in such a prestigious venue by such a prestigious surgeon, filled me with confidence.

I couldn't see a huge difference immediately after the treatment. I thought the effect was OK, but nothing spectacular. But I kept telling myself to wait for a few weeks to see the full effect and to remind myself that it would have cost a lot of money if I had paid for it myself. The appearance of the back of my hands never really did look that different, and in time I almost forgot about the treatment I had allowed myself to have done. Nearly two years later this is the treatment that came back to haunt me.

I had been to a company conference in Rome and the weather had been incredibly hot. I had made the mistake of shaving my bikini line before wearing tight shorts and going out on a bit of a wine bar crawl. Within a day or two I had developed the worst case of itchy weeping spots around my fanny. They were so bad that I ended up in in A and E with severe folliculitis, but slightly troubled that perhaps it might have been a sexually transmitted disease. Thankfully it wasn't, and a course of antibiotics did sort it out. Whilst I was there I pointed out to the doctor that I had some really strange rapid growths appearing on the back of my hands.

She was rather puzzled by these odd growths and the fact that they were very hard. She said I needed further investigation to rule out sarcoidosis (lumps) on the lungs and other vital organs.

I got quite worried after being referred to have CT scans, biopsies, blood tests and other investigations. But after various investigations it was decided that the growths on the back of my hands were in fact a filler-induced granulomatous reaction to the treatment I had had 2 years before. Rare, but not unheard of. There were a few treatment options, including surgery, but the doctors decided to try various medications first.

I had some very painful steroid injections in the back of my hands, and months of antibiotics and oral steroids (which gave me dreadful insomnia). After six months the growths settled down and reduced in size, leaving just a grey hue on the back of both hands. I thought that was it, but the growths came back again not long ago, and I had to have yet another course of treatment. I hope I won't need surgery to cut the growths out, but this may be inevitable.

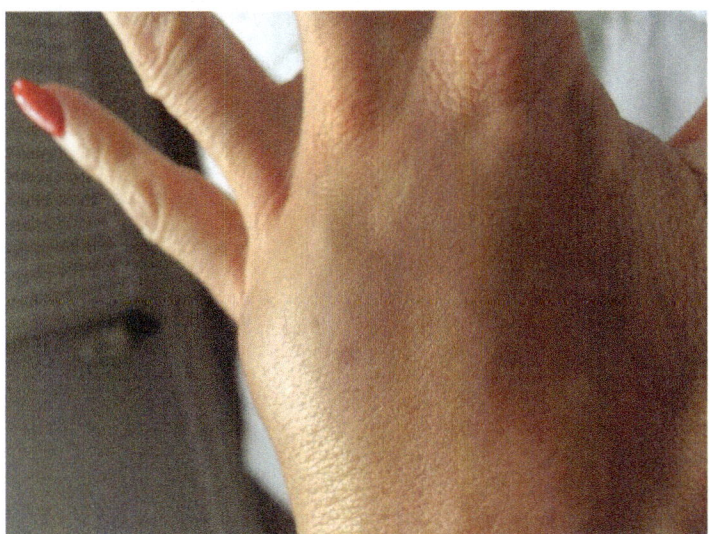

Despite all this, I continue to have Botox (I have my hair back, you understand, and just cannot bear the look of deep frown lines). And I have eyelash extensions, which are utterly ridiculous and very costly. And it goes without saying that I have my nails done regularly with gel which is also very expensive. When your nails grow, which in my case seems to be a few mm each day, there is soon a tell-tale gap emerging between the base of the false nails and your cuticles, and this then needs infilling or your hand looks very unsightly. You can spot women who have gel nails very easily. When I am on the tube I will look at the women sitting opposite me and think to myself how much they need to get infills done urgently.

I keep asking myself, why am I so bothered about what other people think? Why at my age am I not comfortable in my own skin? How come other people seem to be able to just grow older, content that wrinkles and patchy skin are perfectly normal? Other amazing women seem to accept that their waist will probably get a bit bigger and their boobs will probably get a bit saggier, but it is a part of the normal aging process, and it really doesn't matter as long as you have your health.

If someone says to me, gosh you look a bit tired today, or even says that I look well, I still get upset, thinking I must have really bad eye bags, or I think perhaps saying that I am looking well really means I look as if I have put on a bit of weight.

And then I dislike myself even more for caring about remarks that were probably meant to be kind, and there are a billion more important things to be thinking about. And so what if I look tired and I have put a tiny bit of weight on. Why the fuck does that matter so much? It really is pathetic.

Hair-

One question I have asked myself on several occasions is why do I have pathetic thin straight hair on my head, but everywhere else is strong dark coarse growth that is infuriatingly difficult to get rid of? There is of course no answer to this, other than perhaps that it is just genetics. I have kept my hair short with highlights for many years now and just keep my fingers crossed that I do not go bald in my old age. I am uncertain if women can get hair transplants?

As for the hair that infuriatingly keeps growing in other areas of my body, I have tried a great number of hair removal treatments. Out of all of them I think I found fanny waxing the worst in terms of pain level, with lasering my armpits and fanny very much a close second.

Should a woman have pubic hair?

There are so many options and if you are truly a feminist why wouldn't you just let your pubes grow wild and free? Instead of having a landing strip, a Brazilian, a Hollywood, or simply a little trim? My children call it laminate flooring when you are completely hair free down below.

I read recently that pubic hair is fashionable again in the porn industry, but since I shaved mine all off bar leaving a heart shaped patch of hair just for a joke on valentine's day one year– I tend to opt for the laminate flooring. I can't unravel, however, whether this is really my choice or whether it's what the norm is, or whether I am doing it to please men. Surely if a man criticized you for having a perfectly beautiful fanny bush then they are the ones with the problem?

Having said that, if you do have a lot of hair down below it is easier to shave the whole lot off in the shower, though, rather than trying to leave a neat little strip.

I don't know why I am mentioning this but the other night I dreamt that no-matter how many times I shaved my pubes, they would grow back within an hour. I would shave first thing in the morning, but by coffee break they were almost four inches long! Like those novelty candles you blow out, but they keep re-lighting themselves. That would really be a nightmare.

Here are my short reviews on hair removal methods- pain level and success

1. Trimming with small nail scissors – this is the easiest but the results aren't always that brilliant and I am not sure I would want to use this method again after my unfortunate accident in the bath - very

cheap though and usually pain free- level 0 or possibly a 10 if you slice off the end of your labia minora

2. Waxing – and I honestly did persevere with this for several months. You need to leave your hair to grow just enough that you can feel and see some stubble. Never ideal if the day you are due a wax is the day you have a date. Lie on a couch, legs akimbo, which is totally embarrassing and try to keep talking as the hot wax is applied followed by a strip of cloth. The cloth is patted down on the wax before being rather dramatically ripped off.

   To help you deal with the pain, some clever beauticians count down from 3 – but rip off the cloth on 2. This works OK the first time they do it but after that you know what's going to happen next. And the pain is totally excruciating. It does looks good for a while after, providing you don't have any kind of reaction – but then the hair just keeps on coming back. I thought the pain I suffered from each time I went for waxing would get less the more I had the waxing done but it simply never did, so in the end I gave up. Also you should never use if taking Roacutane as the wax will most likely pull the top layer of your skin off along with the hair. Pain level 6, or 10 if you are a wuss like me.

3. Lasering – I tried this after my arm pit hair was successfully removed almost completely after about 8 sessions of torture, and hasn't really come back.

But an arm pit is one thing, fanny lasering is a totally different ball game. And, always a glutton for punishment, I opted for anal hair to be zapped at the same time. (maybe I secretly hoped it might get rid of my piles at the same time). No-pain, no gain as they say. This method is the most undignified of all. Requiring your beautician to see your fanny and arse in all their glory. I have never even looked that closely at my nether regions, and by the 6th time of going she must have known more about my intimate parts than my husband or me ever did. Each time the laser zaps you, you feel intense pain and have to keep telling yourself that it will all be worth it in the end. You try to keep talking to the beautician. Distract yourself by digging your nails in to the palm of your hand or squeezing something as hard as you possibly can. In some ways I am glad this didn't work for me – otherwise I would have laminate flooring down below for the rest of my life and there is something weird about that. Pain level- without a doubt -10.

4. Shaving – still the easiest, most effective, providing your razor isn't blunt, least painful and a very cheap way of removing unwanted pubic hair – well I think so anyway. A lot of people say it makes your hair grow back thicker and quicker but I tend to disagree with that. The hair might look thicker as it

grows back, due to the shape of the end of the hair – but if you never let it grow back because you tend to shave very often, then there's no need to worry? A quick shave in the shower in the morning and Bob's your uncle. A clean -shaved childlike fanny. Simples. And pain level 0 - or maybe a bit higher if you shave your actual flaps by mistake (slight warning here also, as shaving can cause ingrowing hairs, leading to folliculitis as in my pubic nightmare).

5. Hair removal Cream – use a special one for the pubes – don't try to save money by using the same one you use for your moustache, for example! I once did this and I had a massive burn mark over the top of my lips for days. This can work and is cheap, but it's a bit smelly and messy. Pain level 0 – usually unless you are allergic ….

6. Plucking – definitely not recommended for the fanny – OK for a few stray long ones that seem to appear overnight as if by magic. Pain level 3 (weird how as you get old, random hairs just seem to appear anywhere on your body quite literally overnight).

7. Threading – this one originated in Iran/India – best for eyebrows (not even sure if you could do your pubes this way) - basically a cotton thread is twisted and doubled and rolled over the unwanted hair. This plucks the hair out at the follicle level much like using tweezers except on a whole strip of

hair. If it's not done correctly it can be very painful, so I'm giving this a 3-7 on the pain score.
8. Electrolysis – I have never tried this but think I should. It's a method of removing individual hairs from the face or body. The device destroys the growth centre of the hair with chemical or heat energy. After a very fine probe is inserted into the hair follicle, the hair is removed with tweezers. Maybe not so good for the fanny but very possible, and certainly for the bikini area. There is a risk of permanent scarring but I guess that's not bad if it's down below. It can also take up to 12 treatments and up to 2 years to get permanent results. I am reliably told its very painful – but perhaps the results would be worth it?
9. Sugaring - or sugar waxing - or Persian waxing is a method of hair removal that's been used since 1900BC. They probably used honey originally. It's like waxing but it's less painful as the sugar paste doesn't stick to the skin like wax, it only grabs the hair and removes it when pulled. The only issue for me with sugaring is that hair needs to be at least ¼ inch long - so your fanny would be a pretty hairy prickly bush before having this method done.

I had many of these treatments whilst I was married and although I am so much more at peace with myself than I have ever been, I don't think I will ever be free of this desire to be more beautiful than I am, look younger than I am, be thinner than I am.

I even have an app that gives you an estimate of how old you look when you put in a photo - how-old.net - I still do this regularly and get very upset when it says I am older than I actually am. When it comes back with an age that's a lot younger it still makes me happy! That's just ridiculous, I know.

Chapter 6

Leading up to and including my marriage

I haven't said much about my marriage yet but perhaps now is the right time to do so. I really do need first, however, to touch on what happened to me just before I met my ex-husband as this had a profound effect on why I married him and perhaps why I found it so incredibly difficult to leave him.

When I met my ex-husband I was a single mum.

This is what had happened.

One day when my teeth were giving me yet more pain due to the woeful care I used to take of them, the endless bulimia and polo mint sucking, I found myself in Kings College Hospital Dental School, being seen by a tall handsome young dentist. At the time I had a very short skirt on with white knickers that showed every time I bent down - a fact which he told me later was what attracted him to me (well it certainly wasn't my teeth).

After my treatment we arranged to meet up for a drink and I very quickly fell for his charm. And bizarrely his utter desire to have a child with me. I never really wanted children, and thought no-one would ever want children with me, so to have this young handsome man urge me to stop taking contraception, get pregnant and marry him was just mind blowing.

His name was Jacob. He drove a Mazda MX5 red convertible which I thought was utterly amazing. He was tall, blonde, handsome and talented. His parents were, and still are, the most wonderful people I have ever been fortunate to have met, and add to this he said he wanted me, and more than that, he wanted to have a baby with me.

Looking back on my time with Jacob, there was always a nervousness about him. He often made secret phone calls. I once overheard one long call with his brother who is a doctor, discussing Jacob's ex-girlfriend. I learnt later that he was trying to find out if she had got pregnant with his child but had subsequently had an abortion. Ironically she worked in Kings Hospital in the termination clinic. Jacob discovered that she had aborted his child and I always had a feeling that he had got me pregnant simply to prove that he could have a child somehow. This may not be exactly true but there was definitely something in this theory. We had only been together a few months when I found myself pregnant. I was in bed knowing that my period had been late and wondering if I could be pregnant. I decided to take a test. When the blue line appeared I thought – "fuck, am I mad?" Soon after I discovered I was pregnant Jacob asked me to marry him and gave me a (very cheap as it turned out when I pawned it later) engagement ring. Over the next few months I knew that he was in contact with his ex but I never said anything.

When I was around 22 weeks pregnant Jacob said he had changed his mind and wanted to leave me. He asked me if I would consider terminating the pregnancy. This was utterly unthinkable considering I was already showing and the baby was kicking.

I honestly don't know how I got through the rest of the pregnancy. Jacob went back to his ex, who he subsequently married and had 2 children with. They only recently found out that they had a half-sister. I carried on working as long as I could, still maintaining contact with him for some unknown reason. He even came to the birth of my daughter although he had no right to do so. Maybe I was thinking he might change his mind; I really don't know. He only saw our daughter maybe 3 times after that. He left a few bags of nappies outside the front door of my flat a few times and gave me a small amount of money each month for a while.

Two days after my daughter was born I pushed her home from the hospital in a second hand pram. I named her after Charlotte Rampling, an actress I always thought sophisticated but sexy. Home was a flat fairly close to Kings College Hospital and it was annoyingly up 6 flights of stairs without a lift. As I had little money, and being uncertain of whether I would get my job back, I hadn't bought much. She slept, very comfortably I should say, in the bottom drawer of a chest of drawers for a while.

I was very lucky to get my job back and returned to work after 6 weeks. I employed a full-time childminder to care for my daughter and she was the most beautiful contented baby I could wish for. I was just utterly in love with her. Although incredibly tiring I actually found being a single mum was really rewarding and enjoyable. She was, luckily for me, a really good baby. My child minder was wonderful and my job paid enough for me to be able to afford the care I needed. When I was away on conferences, Lottie, as she has always been called by her friends, stayed with my ex's parents, who always loved her and said that in some way they wish their son had married me. On reflection, he never really loved me, and it would never have worked.

When Lottie was about twelve or thirteen, her dad had a terrible car accident. At the time of the accident he had already divorced his wife and he was driving far too fast in his Mazda which overturned. He broke his neck.

It was a terrible accident. He became a paraplegic. And not only did he have no movement below the neck, he was cursed with having endless pain. He wanted to die and every time his parents visited him he begged them to help him to end his life. Whatever I had thought of him was really irrelevant as I would never wish this on anyone.

He passed away earlier this year after the most horrible of existences for fifteen years.

When Lottie was about ten months old I was at work one day, showing some baby photos to a receptionist at one of the doctor's surgeries I used to visit. A young man walked in and complimented them. He ended up being my husband for twenty-one years.

He was new to the pharmaceutical industry and seven years younger than me. He seemed kind and genuinely interested in the photos of Lottie, and he asked me out then and there. There are many bad things I could write about my ex, but I can't forget that he tried to look after me, understand my issues, and he had to go against the wishes of his parents in order to marry me. His dad was Russian and his mum was from Belgium. They weren't conventional and his upbringing certainly wasn't, which I think contributed to his behaviour.

His parents had a list of all the qualities a woman must have if their son was going to marry her, and he couldn't even tick off the first three with me. I am sure there were 10 points and I only scored one, which was that I must be a woman.

1. Be catholic
2. Be younger than him
3. Have no children
4. Be a woman

To my ex-husbands credit, he chose me and Lottie over his parents which I know must have really hurt him at the time. The first day I met John's parents was at a funeral. I was eight months pregnant with our son. John's had a step-brother, who was the son of his Russian father and his father's first wife who was Turkish. He had been married to an Algerian lady. This poor lady had got fed up with his womanizing and she had sadly gassed herself in a car in a garage in Croydon, leaving 2 young children behind. The funeral would have been material for a comedy sketch had it not been so sad. So many nationalities were present that day. The Turkish contingent arrived in 4 black limos all wearing exactly the same black long coats with mobile phones permanently attached to their ears. They looked like security body guards, or the mafia. These phones seemed to go off very regularly including just as the coffin was being lowered in to its grave.

John's family were different. His step-brother once owned a souvenir shop on Oxford Street and always got himself into money problems - which John always sorted out. John also had a younger brother who had Asperger syndrome and was a big drain on the family's time and resources. He had another brother who is incredibly brainy, who seems to have been doing some sort of degree forever, a masters or PHD in Astro Physics; I'm still not certain if even at the age of 40-something that he ever did get any real work, but then I suppose there's not much call for a super brainy astrophysicist. John's nan died of alcoholism and his mum sadly had liver cancer, potentially related to alcohol, and has now also sadly died. He has also struggled with his own alcohol intake and his controlling nature. I mention all of this because it shaped the man he was/is.

I cannot dispute his total love for me and for the kids, but it was twisted and damaged from his upbringing.

I also need to say that he provided for me and the children materially very well indeed. We always had great holidays and we didn't want for much, except perhaps, for a normal life.

He needed to control me. And he wanted sex all the time. I often would just allow him to fuck me to try to put him in a better mood. I struggled to tell him how I really felt, believing being compliant would be the best thing for peace in the home.

He once bought me some pills from the internet which were supposed to make me less frigid and I even took them for a while. But I got hairy and spotty as a result. And I definitely didn't fancy him. I never really did. I had married him because I was scared to be alone and he had asked me. I knew from day one there was something wrong with his attitude to sex and alcohol. Something I should have been able to talk to someone about, to talk to him about, but I just couldn't.

I would always be slightly afraid of what he would do if the children didn't live up to his expectations. They weren't even naughty kids and they weren't stupid either.

They knew when they saw me close to tears many times that I was desperately unhappy.

They also didn't want their dad to know when they had messed up.

I even used to doctor their school reports before I showed them to their dad, tippexing out the bad bits, and re-photocopying them.

I used to love taking the dog out for an hour of space and my son would often come with me to get away from the tense atmosphere at home. We even made up a game. How many ways could we think of killing dad. Blow him up! Hand grenade! Drown him. Push him in front of a train. Poison him. Tie him to a rocket and send him into outer space! Lock him in a ship's container and forget about him. The ways we could kill him became more and more ridiculous.

Looking back I realize how dreadful this was, but it made my son laugh as we tried to release our tension.

After many years with his constant need for sex, and constant controlling behaviour I had to leave. My son was now taller than my husband. One day John had called me pathetic and stupid. I can't remember what I had done but it obviously wasn't good enough. My son overheard the remark and came downstairs, angry and upset. He stood over John and told him in no uncertain terms, "Don't ever talk to mum like that ever again". My son's bravery in standing up to his dad, along with my eldest's support, made me realize that I could, and had to leave.

This was the most harrowing time for me, and for the children.

John couldn't accept that our marriage was over. He kept on pushing me for a reason why I might want to leave him. He said he would even understand if perhaps I had had an affair or had fallen in love with someone else. In the end I made up that I had slept with someone at work, just to try and give him a reason to hate me.

Later he claimed that he had had lots of invasive tests to ensure I had not passed on a sexually transmitted disease to him. When he found out I had made up sleeping with someone, he called the police and said he wanted me arrested for causing him grievous bodily harm.

He wasn't thinking right.

I was actually a bit scared of him during the last few weeks of our marriage as his behaviour was unpredictable. My mum later told me she had called the police four times during that period, worried he might harm me or the children, or do something stupid.

He repeatedly said that he would commit suicide if I left him. He wrote suicide notes and regularly would leave them for me to find, along with a bottle of whiskey and a rope.

He said that when I told him our marriage was over he had googled the height of the local Sainsbury's to find out if he could jump off and kill himself.

One time he even tried to throw himself out of the car as I was driving with Mia in the back. Another time he left to go into the local woods with a rope and a knife and said he was going to hang himself. I called the police. They rang his mobile, which he answered, and then they got him back.

Every time I said I would leave him, he threatened to kill himself. So I stayed as long as I could bear it. Mia said that if he had actually gone through with it she would blame herself for being part of the problem.

Staying in the same house as him was so traumatic. I lost a stone in weight (for once I had actually stopped thinking about food constantly)and found it so hard to keep working, but I had to.

I am not sure exactly when he decided that our marriage was definitely over, but one day he said he would leave and agreed we would put the house on the market.

I organized everything. And after 21 years of marriage there was a lot to sort out. I am not sure how I actually did it, looking back. But the house got sold and he moved out to London having secured a new job. The house sale took ages to go through, though, and I was left with just Mia in the house, using all my savings to pay the mortgage until the sale finally went through.

We got a separation agreement drawn up and agreed to simply go our different ways, splitting the proceeds of the house in half. I realized later to my detriment that I should have got a divorce and a financial settlement agreed from the outset.

Because the house sale had taken so long, I lost the house I was going to buy and had nowhere to live for a bit.

I stayed in a local hotel with Mia for 6 weeks whist I sorted another house out.

The house I eventually bought was a wreck. The lady who once owned it had rented it out to a criminal who had trashed the place before leaving. There were holes in the walls, stains all over the carpets and the kitchen resembled a war zone. The toilets were disgusting. But she wanted a quick sale to get rid of the property, which worked for me.

When I got the keys and the house was officially mine, I stood outside the front door and cried for a long time. Not tears of sadness. Tears of joy and utter relief that finally I was to start a new life, in my own home, on my own terms and he couldn't hurt me anymore.

I employed a builder and his team to gut the place and re-decorate on a budget. I am certain I was ripped off as I handed bundles of cash over to him, having said that the place was fit to live in after just three weeks.

A very good friend of mine cleared all the crap in the garden and took on the project of making it a lovely space to sit out in on warm days. She transformed a weed-ridden wasteland into a small Italian style garden, with rose bushes and a patio.

I loved that house and everything it stood for. My children stayed with me for my very first Christmas not long after I moved in. I am not the best of cooks so I bought everything from M & S. All I needed to do was check the labels for the cooking times and crack open the prosecco.

It was the first Christmas I could remember where there were no arguments. Usually my ex insisted the kids got changed before lunch, whereas I would have been happy if they had stayed in their pyjamas all day. He would also buy "special" presents for them just from him - usually expensive ones like cameras or lap-tops, and then make everyone watch as they opened them.

I remember that first Christmas we played board games all together and for the first time we laughed a lot.

I also remember my eldest and I sitting next to each other whilst we compared potential TINDER dates. I will return to my internet dating later.

Chapter 7

Bucket lists

It was during that time I started writing my bucket lists.

A "life experience" bucket list and a "sexual" bucket list

"Life Experience Bucket List" - in no particular order and some admittedly very boring

1. Learn to Pole Dance/Pole Fitness
2. Go to Ibiza
3. Do Glastonbury
4. Skinny dipping in the sea
5. Try some hash cookies
6. Get a new job
7. Be financially secure
8. Support my youngest daughter's dream to go to Musical Theatre School
9. Give blood
10. Fall in love and meet the man I want to spend the rest of my life with

"Sexual Bucket List"- in no particular order and most definitely not boring!-

1. Threesome – 2 women, 1 man
2. Threesome - 2 men, 1 woman
3. Anal
4. Emmanuel – 2 guys with anal penetration and vagina at same time
5. Holiday romance
6. Dressing up/burlesque
7. Naughty place - (library as per recurring dream)
8. Very young
9. 50 Shades – rough bottom slapping/handcuffing experience
10. The unexpected lover (ie- fat/old/ugly)

Life Experience Bucket List

1. Learn to pole dance
Why the pole? Well, the idea had come from the lady who did my eyelash extensions at the time, which was yet another extravagance and something I am totally addicted to now. She told me that she had tried it and thought I should give it a go. I've always tried to keep fit and enjoyed dancing, and this seemed like the perfect way to keep fit and be sexy at the same time. Since I started pole fitness/dancing there has been a huge increase in the

number of women going to pole classes. It has slightly sleazy connotations to a lot of people, but actually it's a brilliant way to keep fit, meet new people and potentially unleash a sexy side you never knew you had.

As soon as I could, I joined a pole fitness class where I met a group of amazing women. There were women of all shapes and sizes and all abilities: some married, some single and one man – who was actually really good. I found I could invert (that means go upside down) quite easily and had the strength and flexibility to master quite a few moves very quickly. My only downfall is that I bruise easily and am not particularly good with pain.

On many occasions after trying out some new moves or holds during the class I would come home with the most dreadful bruises, looking like I had been in some sort of car accident! I just wanted to learn a new spin or a new pose. We actually had a name for when you mastered a new trick. We called this having a polegasm! I had never giggled so much, swore so much or enjoyed myself so much in ages. I really looked forward to going to classes each week and I actually bought my own pole so that I could practice my holds and moves in between classes. I even had some private lessons at home. I still have my pole up in my bedroom and often when no one is in the house I will play some music really loudly and have a sexy, dirty, sweaty dance around it. I also have been known to put on a sexy Santa fancy dress outfit and give a little special dance just for my partner.

Sadly I am unable to go to classes anymore. This is because I had to have nearly a year off after practically ripping my shoulder out of its joint and, very frustratingly, it has never really recovered. I had a lot of physio and several steroid injections but it still isn't quite right.

Ironically I didn't injure my shoulder doing Pole, but whilst doing a Tough Mudder obstacle course. Even though I can't do the lifts as I did before, the dancing is still fun and I am not quite ready yet to take down the pole. Maybe when I'm sixty. Who knows?

2. Go to Ibiza
On my life list there was a trip to Ibiza. The main thing I wanted to experience was the sunset at Café Mambo. Café Mambo calls itself the ultimate hot spot for the world's most iconic sunset. Delicious food, cocktails and stunning DJ sets. Located in San Marco, I had wanted to go there for years. I just wondered if at fifty two I would be far too old.

I needn't have worried. My friend Claire was, and still is, in love with Ibiza. I used to work with Claire when she was my colleague in the same pharmaceutical company. She had left mainstream pharmaceuticals and was working in a cosmeceutical company selling breast implants to private doctors across London. It made me smile thinking of Claire travelling on the tube with a bag of boobs. These were sample breast implant to show prospective surgeons. She was very familiar with Ibiza and encouraged me to come with her and a group of her friends. She and her friends turned out to be amazing, and some of the strongest women I have ever had the fortune to spend time with. All beautiful, all incredibly intelligent yet funny and all also completely open to new experiences and living their lives to the full. They had all also gone through tough experiences in their lives, and three of us had been through very difficult divorces.

Claire has recently survived cancer, having gone through the experience and treatment with such amazing bravery. This is typical of her nature and attitude of never giving up. Claire believed in living life to the full, even before her cancer. She really loves techno/house music and dance music in general. She had been to many of the clubs in Ibiza on several occasions and just gave me the confidence to go and have some fun, no matter what my age was.

Denise was the only woman slightly older than me, and she was the most amazing story teller. And she had some amazing stories to tell. We would sit on the beach with bottles of wine, plastic glasses and nibbles at the ready, and listen to her describe some of the fabulous things she had done. These included making wigs for Cher and Kylie Minogue, dating Christopher Reeve AKA Superman, meeting Roger Federer, and so much more. She now has a hugely successful company in medical tattooing, Some of it cosmetic and some compassionate for women who have received life changing injuries, for example, through horrendous acid attacks Sam was beautiful and vivacious. Her son is a lead musician in a band who were doing a season in Ibiza that summer. He got us all on the guest lists of all the major clubs on the Island. She was funny and very generous spirited.

Angie ran her own highly successful business and travels all over the world promoting her women's health products. She was the more calming influence on our group and the only one with a successful marriage as it happens.

Asa was the youngest. She was a dentist with a smile to match and just about everyone, or every man we met, instantly fell in love with her. If she had wanted to she could have easily slept with a different guy every single night. But she didn't. She was dating a man she had met on the internet and seemed to have fallen for him very quickly. She would spend hours talking to him each day on the phone. I think he was keeping tabs on her and worried she might meet someone else.

The week we were in Ibiza I didn't get much sleep. I did fulfil my dream of watching the most beautiful sunset from Café Mambo - whilst smoking a shisha pipe. I watched dancers and jugglers on the beach and everyone seemed incredibly happy. As the sun finally set to the sound of Enya singing Sail Away, everyone watching spontaneously burst in to a round of applause. It was very surreal but every bit as good as I had hoped it would be.

As far as the night clubbing went we went clubbing five days in a row. We went to Amnesia first. This was once the estate of a wealthy Spanish family. It has two rooms and an "ice cannon". Completely crazy atmosphere with everyone dancing and drinking and many, no doubt, taking something they should not have done.

DC-10 was another nightclub but not my favourite, as I stood out like a sore thumb in a lace mini-dress. It is an old converted estate right near the airport runway. They play heavy techno music with laser light shows and definitely suited to a younger crowd. Pa T cha, in Ibiza Town, was more my style and although they have a 'Fuck Me I'm crowds Famous' Thursday night, I didn't meet anyone famous there, didn't get fucked and for whatever reason I got approached by several people that night to ask me if I had any drugs they could buy (I either "looked" like a dealer, or was so much older than most there it must have been assumed I was). Space Ibiza was fun, a mega-club hot spot and one of the oldest and largest clubs. We went there after a brilliant evening at Ushuaia. Ushuaia is an open air beachside party spot. Kygo was playing there the night we went and I danced all night, quite a lot of the time in the pool, wearing a string swimming costume and heels. I didn't take any drugs and I didn't sleep with anyone.

I did go topless in Ibiza for pretty much the first time ever and I got absolutely plastered on a beach after drinking some very interesting shots of a clear liqueur. I remember nearly getting decapitated by a ceiling fan after jumping on a table in a bar to dance to a band playing there. I am sure the sight of a fifty plus woman going crazy, tits flying all over the place, was not a pretty one.

Ah well, at least number two was ticked off that bucket list.

3. Glastonbury

Doing Glastonbury. Bearing in mind I hate camping, have very private toilet habits and like to wash my hair every day, this was only ever going to turn out badly.

I have many friends who absolutely love Glastonbury and can't wait to get tickets each year. Getting tickets is a feat in itself, because as soon as they become available just about the whole of the UK are dialling in to see if they can get some. So many people miss out but I was lucky and managed to get tickets for a group of five.

The year I went, sadly the weather was mediocre. Not a complete wash out – but plenty of mud and bloody freezing at night. I went with Claire and three of her festival friends. If you have ever been to Glastonbury music festival you will know the horrendous queues to get in to the site and then having to trudge for about 2 hours dragging all your stuff to get to your pitch.

Exhausting to say the least.

Then the problems really start if you need a pee or a poo. You can't simply just drop your jeans down and squat as this is not allowed due to environmental reasons. If everyone pissed on the land it would have destroyed it. If you need a wee, girls can use a plastic "ladies urinal funnel" or shewee and wee in to a bottle or bucket. The wee would have to be disposed of later. If a shewee doesn't appeal then you can always go to "the long drop". I have nightmares about the long drop. Using the long drop is bad enough if you need a pee but absolutely horrendous if you need a shit. The long drops are rows of cubicles, with a kind of loo seat in each cubicle and a hole beneath each seat leading to a deep chasm of shit and piss and loo paper beneath. The cubicles had ¾ size doors so you could see peoples' feet below the doors from outside and potentially their heads above the doors. The long drops were, of course, unisex which added an extra bit of smelly fun.

I actually can't remember if there was a loo seat the first time I went in to a cubicle because I was so traumatized. I remember squatting and trying really hard to do a poo but it just wasn't going to happen whilst I was there. All I ever managed to release was a rather embarrassingly loud fart. I am usually pretty regular but trust me I did not manage a single little plop any one of the five days I was there. All that backed up shit had to eventually come out – and when it did it was more painful to start with than giving birth. Apart from not shitting, I also didn't shower or wash my hair as the shower block was miles away and I couldn't bear the walk of shame to get to it. So I used baby wipes and boiled a kettle in the tent and used that water to wash my face. I bought a crazy pink felt hat with a large flower attached to the brim and wore it all week.

The shewee I had bought before going was very useful at night as I could pee into a bottle and then dispose of it in the morning.

My Glastonbury experience definitely wasn't anything like the one Bridget Jones had. I definitely didn't meet a gorgeous looking millionaire who I had incredible sex with on a double bed in a yurt! Although I did actually fall flat on my face in the mud dragging my slightly broken trolley loaded with all my camping stuff though miles of fields on the way from my car to our pitch.

Despite all the bad experiences I had at Glastonbury, the music and the camaraderie were great and I saw a lot of fantastic bands, including Coldplay, Adele, Muse, James Blake and so many more. The silent disco was hilarious as well. Everyone wore headphones and danced to a choice of four sound tracks which meant that we were all dancing to a different beat. We did that on the first day when I felt and smelt relatively human.

There was so much to see, listen to, experience, eat, drink, and in my opinion there were almost too many stages and exhibits. And despite my best planning and trudging around in muddy wellies from stage to stage I barely got to see half of what I intended to.

Coldplay were the final act and they finished playing at around midnight on the last day. I had to get back home as I was meant to be catching a flight to Switzerland the next morning for some company training. But I got lost trying to find my way back to my car and it took over two hours to find it. By the time I found my car I was desperate for a wee. I simply couldn't be arsed if anyone saw me so I simply got the shewee out in the car park and pulled down my jeans to go in full view of everyone. Unfortunately I missed the funnel and peed all down my legs and shoes. As my jeans were soaked in piss and I was really, really tired I decided to simply just whip everything off, have a quick clean with a baby wipe, pull on some pyjama bottoms that were conveniently at the top of my bag and grab a pair of flip-flops to complete the outfit.

Bearing in mind I was still wearing my pink felt hat, the look was totally ridiculous to say the least, and slightly embarrassing when I had to stop for petrol at about 4 am in the morning on the long tedious drive back. I got home in the morning around 6:30 am, slept for two hours and then had to get up to go to the airport for my flight. I have no idea how I managed to make it.

I won't be going back to Glastonbury any time soon, but at least I fulfilled number three on my bucket list.

As for the other items, I am still to skinny dip in the sea (although technically I was naked in the sea once in Corfu, having a shag with an old boyfriend when a passing cruise boat full of tourists guessed what was going on and gave us a loud cheer and a round of applause). I am still not sure that I am financially secure – but all the rest I have done.

Chapter 8

Internet dating

So it is time to talk about my "sexual bucket list" and the on-line dating that led me to achieving it.

When you have been married to the same person for twenty-one years and are in your fifties, internet dating can be a really daunting and very scary thought. But when all your friends are either married or in a long term relationship it can be potentially the best way to meet new people and definitely worth considering.

All three of my children are Tinder experts which is the most popular App used, partly because its free and partly because it is so easy.

I was definitely open to the idea of it, but I was very much less certain about how I should behave if and when I first met any of the potential dates. Despite all my reservations I decided to sign up to a few agencies and see what happened.

These are the few I tried:

Match.com - online dating service with web sites serving over 50 countries in twelve languages. You can pay for different plans, just for a month or six months which works out a lot cheaper if you don't meet someone during the first month. Every day Match.com brings matches straight to your inbox. You can have a quick check to see if you might be interested in meeting any of them. I think there a few fake profiles, but I'm not entirely sure.

Elite Singles - supposedly focused on pairing up singles who are not only matched intellectually, but also financially. It is supposed to be a really good site for mature and educated professionals. Some reviews give this 4.5 out of 5 but others only a 1 star which is the rating I would have given it when I tried it.

eHarmony – they say they deliver better dates. And claim that every 14 minutes someone finds love on eHarmony. You can join for free, but all the photos are blurry until you upgrade to a paid account. And it is relatively quite expensive.

P.O.F (plenty of fish) – over 90 million people use POF. Its free and you can contact members without paying. The problem I found with POF was that a lot of the men that used it seemed to use it as a platform for sex. I certainly got a lot of dick pics from guys using POF. Perhaps its reputation is well founded

Tinder – This is the world's most popular app for meeting new people. It apparently has 30 billion matches to date. It is basically a location-based networking and online dating app that allows users to anonymously swipe to like or dislike other profiles based on their photos, a small bio, and common interests. Once two users have "matched" they can exchange messages.

Happn – explained in a bit

Other sites I have not tried include-

Mysinglefriend.com - this is the only online dating site that puts your friends in charge of your profile. It is safe, secure and anonymous. You chose a username and set up a profile describing yourself and the type of person and relationship you are looking for. I am not sure I would want my friends in charge of my profile.

Zoosk - This site claims to connect compatible people and constantly improves matches by "studying" users' behaviour.

Ourtime - for meeting like-minded singles over 50

Pin-flirt – this is for flings and hook ups with no strings attached

The funniest thing, or perhaps the most irritating thing I should say, was when I got matched twice to my ex-husband. This was when I was using Match.com and when I used eHarmony. I might sound a bit cruel but the way he described himself seemed very conceited to me – he genuinely believed he was quite a catch and thought his profile would impress any possible future dates.

Setting up your profile on any of these sites and deciding which photos of yourself to use is actually really difficult and after meeting a few men it certainly seems to me that men exaggerate all their so-called best qualities, which often included the size of their dicks if you were using some of the free sites. I must have had dozens of dick pics sent to me which were somehow meant to impress me and make me want to meet the men they belonged to. I guess some women might have enjoyed them but I certainly didn't.

I had the least success with the most expensive dating site that I tried, which at the time was Elite Singles. The questionnaire I had to fill out to personalize my profile and give me more of a chance of meeting someone compatible was unbearably long and in the end turned out to be totally useless. I got matched with guys who lived half the country away, were far too old, and also with men who smoked, even though I had said I didn't want to meet a smoker. That was a huge waste of my money and my time, and I got charged for an extra 6 months because I forgot to cancel my subscription in time. Please be careful and definitely read the small print if you decide to pay a subscription, and remember to cancel it when it doesn't work out for you. Having said that it didn't work for me, a very good friend of mine met her current husband through Elite Singles and is really happy, so maybe it was just me.

The first date, and in fact most of the dates I went on, was when I was using the site called "Happn" At the time it was quite a London centric dating app and because I worked in London, I met a lot of men through this app.

Happn is a location-based social search mobile app that allows users to like or dislike other users, and allows users to chat if both parties like each other. It's free, which is a good start and it uses your GPS location to search within a 250 meter radius of where you are and will show you other Happn users in the same area. It doesn't show you profiles of anyone you haven't crossed paths with.

Because London is so diverse and such a big melting pot of nationalities, I met many men from so many different countries. It was only when I considered writing this book that I realized I had done a Lisa Stansfield – and been "All around the world" so to speak (mainly Europe I guess though).

So let's see -here is a list of some of those who I met and who helped me complete my sexual bucket list - this is by no means an exhaustive list, but it certainly was exhausting. I won't go through all of the dates, just some of the more memorable ones.

The Gorgeous Geek Cypriot
The Italian Gold dealer
The Canadian Pilot
The German Sports Reporter
The Irish Millionaire

The English Eccentric
The naughty troubled Northerner
The Asian Businessman
The Egyptian Egotist
The saucy Spaniard
The Member of Parliament
The Italian Stallions (although one was more like a pony to be fair)
The Cockney Rebel
The French Philosopher – he liked to read poetry to me but we never actually met
The Responsible Russian – we met once, I got very drunk and missed my last train home. He paid for me to stay in a suite at the Renaissance hotel after declining sex due to lack of a condom. He then had an accident on his way home, breaking his arm, and we never met again.

Contacting potential dates. So easy to get it very wrong.

When I first started up a text conversation with a potential new date, I really had no idea of what "texting" behaviour I should adopt.

I simply had no idea about the dos and don'ts of texting potential new partners. My kids were absolutely appalled at what they considered to be my total and utterly inappropriate texting behaviour. When I got a text from a potential date I would get ridiculously excited, and act like a stupid teenager. As soon as my phone beeped and I saw that I had a message I could not control myself and simply had to read the message immediately, and then reply immediately (whilst ridiculously as it sounds now, I'd be giggling and silently screaming - oh my god, oh my god, I think he really likes me).

Apparently, the etiquette you have to follow is that you must not read the text when it first arrives, however painful that may feel, even if you know you have got one from someone you really fancy. You must not read the message for at least an hour. And then, once you have read it, do not reply immediately. The reasoning is that you do not want the man to feel that you might be too intense or too needy. The funny thing was that at first I wasn't actually looking for a long term relationship at all. After all I had just come out of a twenty-one year nightmare one, where sex was a chore and I got told how to behave.

I was initially just looking for fun and an opportunity to try things out that I had never done before. I was up for meeting anyone who was vaguely attractive and ideally not too old. Also, preferably and unashamedly at the time, with some money to spoil me.

I think there are a lot of men who are on these sites, or at least in my experience, who are just looking for fun and definitely not for a long term relationship, whereas the majority of women, I am told, are looking for that "special" someone to spend the rest of their life with. I think one of the reasons I had such a good or interesting experience of internet dating was because I wasn't looking for hubby number two, at least not at the beginning.

Back to the text etiquette, another issue about texts was deciding when and if to put a kiss or an emoji at the end. Should I wait till they put kisses on their messages before I ended mine with a kiss, and also did I need to worry if the kisses came too soon and there are were too many.

Just getting the text conversations right before I went on a first date was a nightmare, let alone any phone calls. In fact, as strange as it may seem, on many occasions I would meet someone for the first time without even having had a phone conversation with them. It was all done by text and then I would meet them somewhere in a mutually agreed location which was very often in a London bar.

I now wonder if the Booking Office Bar at St Pancras thought I was a high class prostitute as I nearly always arranged my first date there, and with a different man, on so many occasions. It wasn't long before the staff there would welcome me by name and find me a table, probably wondering who I might be meeting and why.

Many things would run through my mind when deciding how to behave on the first date. There are also rules, of course, about how many times you should meet a guy before sleeping with him. I did try hard at first to adhere to the "at least twice" rule but then quickly decided to abandon the rules if and when I met a seriously hot guy, and especially if I had drunk a whole bottle of prosecco. I recently heard Janet Street-Porter say on Loose Women that she would always sleep with her date on the first night, and then if they were crap in bed she didn't have to bother seeing them again.

If the rules, however, were likely to be broken, I had to ensure that I was fully prepared in more ways than one.

- Any evidence of any bodily hair in the wrong place must be removed by whatever means suitable (feel free to refer back to my hair removing chapter!)
- Get nails done so they look immaculate (definitely no tell-tale infill gap)
- Eyelash extensions done the day before
- Get on the cross trainer or in the gym that afternoon
- Try to have a shit before the date – nothing worse than needing to have a shit on a first date (either before bed, or in the morning)
- Don't eat anything that is likely to make you fart
- Don't eat dinner, so your stomach will be as flat as possible
- Wear matching underwear (or none at all)
- Minimum essentials apart from usual makeup bits - Femfresh spray (great fanny/arse deodorant), foldable toothbrush, small mirror, foundation
- Condom – although I have to admit I didn't insist on one all the time. I did, however, get myself checked when I met my current partner, and got the all clear.
- Shaver – just in case a trip to the loo before or after revealed any unwanted pubes or armpit hair

I would go to extraordinary lengths before I went on a first date, just to try to be this perfect version of myself, that was in fact so flawed.

When spending the night with someone for the first time I found it incredibly difficult to relax, which is where the prosecco usually came in particular handy. I couldn't bear the thought of the guy seeing what I really looked like in the morning, especially if I liked him. I would do anything to avoid being seen without make up, and would very often sleep with a full face of makeup on as I was simply too embarrassed for my disgusting skin to be seen by anyone.

When sleeping next to someone for the first time I would try to lie in the best position possible so that my hair would look reasonable in the morning and also make sure my face wasn't pressed too hard against the pillow so as not to disturb any make up that I had left on or to leave any embarrassing makeup stains on the pillow

The other thing that crippled me with embarrassment was the possibility of letting out a noisy or stinky fart. I do tend to fart overnight, or in the morning, especially when building up to a shit. This may be fairly normal, but I felt that I just couldn't let one go within smelling and/or hearing distance of any date, especially on the first meeting.

So I found a way to avoid the embarrassment of an escaping fart. This was by wrapping a bit of loo paper around my middle finger and pressing it hard against my bum hole whilst letting out the fart very, very slowly, thereby hopefully resulting in the fart not being heard or smelt. I would follow this little ritual by using a squirt of Femfresh and a spray of Channel no 5 and then with any luck no guy ever found out.

Looking back on this it all seems so ridiculous. Although many of the men I met cared what they looked like on the first date, and had obviously taken time and trouble about their appearances, I'm certain they didn't care about the odd stray hair or bodily odour. They certainly didn't care about farting or having a dump in the morning.

The complete opposite was true for me, and I think because I didn't want to go for an embarrassing poo in the morning, eventually I actually stopped being able to go at all in the morning. This I truly believed really mucked up my digestive system for a while.

When I started internet dating, I think like a few people who use these sites do, I had a few chats and potential dates on the go at any one time. This meant I could hedge my bets around potential future partners. If, after I met someone who I had been messaging, they turned out to be a complete idiot, I would still be able to meet with someone else that I had been talking to.

I was not very good at this, though, and sometimes it was awkward if I forgot to turn my phone off when with a guy for the first time, and an explicit WhatsApp popped up from someone else.

I decided it was a bit easier to try one date at a time.

Frustratingly, I did meet a lot of men who turned out to be so utterly different from their profiles that as soon as they even entered the bar I knew I had to get away. I would use an excuse like one of my parents had been rushed to hospital, or my daughter had crashed her car, so that I could get away as soon as possible.

I do remember meeting this guy who had sent me endless messages about how he would spoil me with the best champagne, book us on first class tickets to New York, change my life forever and so forth. His picture didn't look too bad and his messages, apart from being a bit full on, were quite exciting. I do remember him saying how fantastic he was in bed and how he would be able to satisfy my every need. That should really have put me off I guess.

The one and only time I met him was in the foyer of the Shard in London. Or rather, this was when I first met his nose, which is possibly the biggest nose I have ever seen in my entire life. Huge. Massive. Gargantuan. Like half his face was actually made up of his nose. Long and curved and so enormous it could have been out of a comedy sketch. He had only put photos of his head facing forward on his profile picture, for obvious reasons. He was also much shorter than he had stated, more like 5ft 2 ins instead of the 5ft 8 ins he had put on his profile.

How would you even snog a guy like this? When I started talking to him I simply could not take my eyes off his nose. It was like I was hypnotized by it. I felt so cruel and shallow but it was a complete turn off and I made my excuses and got out of there in a hurry.

One guy I met told me to meet him at his gym which was close to a tube station near where he lived. I can't remember which tube station this was, but the gym was a good 15 minute walk.

I had made quite a big effort and dressed up as he said we would be going out to dinner. I was wearing the little black dress, high heels and stockings. But that night the weather was miserable, the rain was lashing it down and the wind was howling. It seemed to take me forever to walk to this gym, and I was freezing cold and soaked through, and by the time I got there my umbrella had blown inside out several times.

When he eventually came out of the gym he hadn't even bothered showering and was still in his sweaty gym kit. He barely made eye contact with me and then said, "Right, let's go and pick up a kebab and take it back to my place, I'm fucking starving". Nice.

That night ended abruptly, too, and certainly no opportunity to tick off one of my sexual fantasies.

The first successful date I had after my marriage breakdown was with a man I ended up seeing a few times. He was a rather handsome Greek Cypriot called Demitris. We first met in a very swanky lounge bar on Berkley Street in Mayfair. It was a place I had been recommended to go to by a good friend of mine who loved the atmosphere and clientele who frequented it.

I will say straight away that Demitris was married and he told me this pretty much from the word go. All too often too many of the men I met were already married and Demitris, like a lot of the married men I met, said they would leave their wives if it wasn't for their children. I know that I should not have dated him. It was wrong. Many of the men I met who were married said they were seeking fun with no strings attached and were happy to spoil me on the nights we went out together.

The way I justified my poor behaviour to myself at the time was believing that they were locked in loveless marriages, forced to sleep in separate bedrooms, couldn't leave their wives for fear of losing access to their children and I was providing them with some much needed relief.

Demitris would say things like, "well, a man's got to eat – and when you aren't getting anything at home you have no choice".

He said his wife knew and accepted that his trips to London were for him, basically, to get laid, and as long as he was careful, always came back to her and provided well for her and the kids, that's all that mattered to her, and she would turn a blind eye to his infidelity.

I know I should have told him to fuck off. But he was honest right from the start. He had such charisma. He was tall, handsome and very funny. There was an undeniable chemistry between us and I loved the way he flattered me and spoilt me. I never paid for a thing. He always paid in cash, even when paying hotel bills. He carried a lot of cash.

He was a regular in a hotel in Chelsea and always got the penthouse suite.

For some reason I convinced myself that there was nothing wrong with what he and I were doing, and I accepted his excuses for being secretive, cheating on his wife and never introducing me to anyone he knew.

He was the first person I slept with after I left my ex-husband. It was quite ironic looking back on it now, but I had been with a man for twenty-one years who couldn't last more than a few minutes and now I was with a man who could keep going for ever and very often not even climax. I'm not sure what was worse!

But at least I wanted to be with Demitris and I could do this on my terms.

Or so I thought. Because really, this thing we had, whatever you want to call it, was always on his terms. He would always dictate when and where we could meet. I was always waiting for his texts, ready to drop everything just to fit in to his agenda and I thought I was the one in control.

He sent me links to certain songs and as I listened to them I would believe every word the singer was saying – as if it was Demetris's words to me. Songs like, "Don't look any further" by Dennis Edwards (great song by the way) and another classic "Outstanding" by the Gap Band. I was hooked for a while by his charm, but after he cancelled me on several occasions when he said that he couldn't leave his wife or some other excuse I realized that I was just living in Fantasy Land and that this relationship if you can call it that, was never going to go anywhere.

So, I went back on the Happn app.

I was excited when my path crossed with a good looking youngish man and we both gave each other a heart, indicating we both liked each other.

He was an Italian businessman called Marco. I liked Marco even before I met him He clearly hadn't read the book about texting as he answered nearly all of my messages within a few minutes of receiving them and was soon putting kisses at the end of each of his replies. We finally met in person in the Booking Office and when I walked in he had a huge grin on his face. Tall, dark and, yes, handsome, I knew that the rule of at least two dates before sleeping with someone you have just met was going to go right out of the window. He was genuinely very sweet and certainly seemed to like me a lot. This time he wasn't married, but had recently split with his wife and had two very young children that stayed with him in his flat every other weekend. After a brilliant evening of suggestive chatter and flirting outrageously he asked me not to go home. He made a phone call and we were soon booked in to the Great Northern Hotel; a gorgeous boutique hotel with beautiful wood panelled rooms, hand crafted furniture and gloriously comfortable Hypnos beds. I was very glad I had made all the necessary preparations including bringing a bag of small essential items, just in case. It was a champagne filled fun night and I went home on a high the next morning.

I saw him on quite a few occasions after that, but I never went back to his flat and always saw him in hotels. He was a broker in the city so he could always afford the best hotels and the loveliest restaurants. He was only forty and bearing in mind I was fifty two, I felt too old for him, however exciting it all was.

I did see him one or two times over the next couple of years and he was the last man I slept with before realizing I didn't want to go on with fleeting meaningless relationships anymore. I don't know what it is about Italians but the ones I met all seemed to want to have anal sex.

Marco was no exception and asked me if I was in to it. I was as honest as I could be and told him that it was something I wanted to try. And as this was actually on my sexual bucket list, I had done a bit of research over a few glasses of wine with a gay friend of mine about what the best way to have anal sex for the first time was. It was one of the most hilarious conversations I had ever had. He said it was clearly important to fancy the guy you were going to do the deed with, and be as relaxed as possible. Preferably the guy wouldn't have a huge cock as this could be problematic for the first time. Marco was pretty average in terms of cock size so that was a bit of a relief, and I definitely fancied him so I thought he would be just the right person to try it with. My gay friend had said to me, lube, lube and more lube, was the way to go the first time. Lying on your back with knees up a little would be the best position apparently and also it was important that once you were ready for penetration the guy should just hold the end of his cock in your bum hole first before actually starting to thrust back and forth.

I took all of my gay friend's advice on board and actually found I enjoyed the experience much more than I had expected. And that was a successful tick off the bucket list.

Following the initial dates I had with Marco, and starting to think that hotel shagging was getting a bit boring, I wondered who else might be out there. Not long after meeting Marco I crossed paths with a tall blonde-haired, extremely good-looking German sports reporter. I had been messaging him for a while but we didn't meet for weeks as he was in Germany, where he was building himself a cottage in the countryside that he promised to take me to one day, although he never did.

Magnus and I met periodically on and off for quite a few months. He was actually single, which made a change, and he had a flat near Notting Hill, where I would stay the night. He was ten years younger than me and I knew that to him we were only ever going to be a bit of fun. I thought that a bit of fun was all I needed, but in truth I really did want a bit more than that. Magnus was not particularly romantic and I was endlessly disappointed by the lack of kisses at the end of his messages, and how rarely he ever paid me compliments.

We did however have many good times and I got quite a kick going out with him - even though once again I never got to meet any of his friends. I don't know why I accepted this; in fact, I never even questioned it. Maybe it was because he was young and so good looking. He did have a great arse, however, which I believe resulted from the very unusual way he would have sex. He liked to be on top and squat over me like a frog. I'm sure all of that squatting must have been the reason for that great arse, he certainly didn't seem to do any other type of exercise!

I made the decision to end it with Magnus after eventually I had a good talk with myself about the one-sided nature of our relationship. I think Magnus said that he was sorry I felt like I did, but he couldn't give me any more than he was giving me already.

After Magnus came the Canadian, TJ. TJ was not particularly good looking. He was very slim which I am not attracted to as I am not a fan of hugging someone and being able to feel their bones at the same time. But he had his plus points. He was head of some digital company and also a pilot. He had a place in New York and another in London. Somehow I never got to see either. Although I did have a few amazing dinners in the best restaurants and we did stay in some lovely hotels. The first night we met I had sworn to myself I was going to be good and try to be elegant and sophisticated. That lasted about five minutes. I met him in a grand art deco French brasserie on Sherwood Street, near Piccadilly Circus tube station.

I would definitely recommend going there. It has a really spectacular 1930s original interior. It's not too expensive and every evening there is live music.

I got totally swept away by his accent and the fact that all the waiters seemed to know him. I hadn't eaten anything all day in the vain attempt to have a flat stomach in this skimpy black dress I had worn that night. Wine arrived almost as soon as we sat down and I took a large swig to steady my nerves. He ordered for me which, in hind sight, was probably a bad thing as I didn't like anything that arrived. And as I hadn't eaten anything all day I got totally and utterly pissed very, very quickly indeed. I actually had to go to the loo to be sick (and this had nothing to do with my bulimia) Thankfully, because I was so well practiced in being secretly sick, I just about got away with it. I did have my trusty travel toothbrush and breath freshener in my handbag just in case I needed it. Another woman in the loo asked me if I was alright, and I think I replied by saying, "I think I might be pregnant". She wasn't at all impressed.

When I returned to the table I carried on as if nothing had happened, only to realize a couple of hours later I had missed my last train home. There was no point in me trying to be good at that point, and in any case I was barely even able to walk. I ended up staying with him in a nearby hotel that night; I am sure that the sex was terrible, and I do remember leaving him in bed the following morning to get the first train back home. As all the daily London commuters piled off the train at St Pancras to head for the tube, there was I in my makeup and clothes from the night before, ridiculous heels and mini dress, making the walk of shame down the platform to try and get a seat where no-one could see me. But I am certain they all knew exactly what I had been up to.

I actually had to take two days off work following that night out. I had such a bad hangover I couldn't even take a sip of water without heaving up bile. The hangover from hell meant there was no way that I could have even coped with work. Apart from making myself ill and completely embarrassing myself, another really annoying thing was that I had ruined the heels of yet another brand new pair of shoes. I seemed to be quite good at this as the underground escalators are definitely not designed for thin high heels. I tried to convince myself this would never happen again.

The next rather unfortunate date was with an Asian business man called Lee. His messages had seemed quite normal and he seemed really keen to meet. Almost too keen. He lived in South London and asked that we meet in a pub near where he lived. Lee looked very handsome and sounded like he was quite wealthy. He talked about having a flat, and a large house in the country. I went through my usual routine of getting ready and wondered how this date would go. I arrived before him in the pub he had suggested, which annoyed me a bit considering he was so keen to meet, and had been very specific about the day and time. He was nearly an hour late and I had almost given up on him but he finally rushed in very apologetically, and said he'd make it up to me. He said that that he had some very important family matters he had to deal with.

He said that rather than have another drink there, we should take a drive in to the country as it was such a beautiful evening, and for some reason I agreed. He said it would be good to get out of London and that he wanted to show me his house. The drive seemed to take forever and I began to get a little nervous. We stopped for some petrol and he came back after he had paid, holding a bunch of flowers and a kinder egg of all things. I said that was so sweet of him, but Lee simply muttered that actually they were for someone else.

I realized my mobile had no signal and I was by this time getting very worried. I was starting to think how I might open the car door and throw myself out, when finally we slowed down. We turned in to this gated drive, and the gates opened for us automatically. We drove up this long path to an amazing looking house where there were several other parked cars.

We parked up and he said there was someone he would like me to meet. We walked up to the house; he had the flowers in one hand and the kinder egg in the other. He took me in to a large reception room where there were about twenty people surrounding a bed. In the bed was a very poorly looking old lady. He bent over and kissed her forehead. "Hi, Mum," he said. This is my girlfriend (pointing to me). I've bought you flowers and a little chocolate egg.

I have to admit this was the last thing I was expecting and I was completely lost for words. Everyone was so pleased to meet me and I felt I couldn't say that this was our first date. It seemed like his mother's dying wish was to see him with a nice girlfriend. I wonder now if he was gay to be honest, and perhaps his mum never knew. After the really bizarre start to the evening, worse was to come when around fifteen minutes later the old lady actually died.

Rather than everyone going in to a mad panic and calling an ambulance, this was clearly not unexpected as there was a doctor present and there had been lots of praying going on. What would you have done in these circumstances? In a ridiculous attempt to do something helpful I found the kitchen and made everyone a cup of tea.

Afterwards I called a taxi and politely made my exit. I did not hear from Lee again, and nor did I want to. That was one of the strangest first dates I have ever had.

Time to tick off some more of that sexual bucket list. And this came about through another Italian who, unbelievably, as I discovered later, was a gold dealer. Yes, he actually was a gold dealer. He was called Giovanni, and he lived in four storey house, near Camden.

As for a lot of my dates, I met him via Happn. I wasn't at all sure he would be my type, but his messages were very warm and he wasn't smutty at all. He sounded like he just wanted to have fun. His profile pictures included him having dinner with beautiful friends in beautiful restaurants and I thought I might enjoy being spoiled.

He suggested we went to Novikov's – which definitely worked for me. I made my usual preparations and got the high speed to St Pancras. He was waiting for me there and we jumped into a cab together to go to Mayfair. When I met Giovanni I thought that sadly he wasn't my type at all. He was shorter than me, and a little overweight, but he did have a cheeky smile, a great accent, and he wanted to buy me vodka and champagne. When we got out of the cab there was a huge queue waiting to get into Novikov's, but Giovanni just went straight to the front and said something to the doorman. A few minutes later, as if by magic, we were ushered straight in. The manager of the Italian restaurant, and a lot of the staff at Novikov's, seemed to know him very well. Novikov's is a very glamorous place and owned by Russian entrepreneur, Arkady Novikov, a personal friend, apparently, of Vladimir Putin. There always seemed to be lots of dodgy looking Russian men in the lounge bar downstairs, and a lot of very young beautiful women with them. I wondered if they were high class prostitutes. I didn't care, though, because I loved the vibe in that bar. Fantastic music, low comfy seats, subtle lighting and, most importantly, lots of vodka. While we got to know each other he introduced me to a friend of his who I found out later was a celebrity hairdresser, and also Italian. He was young and very good looking and I couldn't help but fancy him. I also definitely felt the attraction was mutual.

I realized later that the introduction was very deliberate because what followed after that evening, I am convinced was a plan, and had happened before.

Giovanni clearly had a very busy London nightlife. After we left Novikov's we went to a night club which I honestly can't remember the name of. Again, Giovanni seemed to be well known there and immediately the management let us in past the long queue of people waiting to get in. We were taken to our private, roped off seating area and a large ice bucket complete with several bottles of champagne and sparklers was immediately brought to us. By this time I was reasonably squiffy and just completely amazed that I was here and that this was happening + to me, a fifty two year old in a nightclub, drinking champagne with an Italian I had only just met.

We got back to Giovanni's house at around 3am and had some very unmemorable sex. I had a massive hangover in the morning and struggled to process what had happened the night before. I didn't feel like me at all, but despite the conversations I was having in my head about the rights and wrongs of it all, I just knew I wanted to see him and Francesco again. Giovanni had been really nice during the evening and in the morning he even cooked me breakfast which was kind of weird. He questioned me about Francesco, the young Italian he had introduced me to the night before. He wasn't stupid, and knew I fancied him, which was what he wanted to hear I think. He suggested the three of us had dinner together in his house the following week. He never explicitly said, 'are you up for a threesome', but I just knew that was what he was implying.

Once again I had to do the walk of shame at the station that morning, but despite the hangover I also had this feeling of excitement about what might happen the following week. I had quite a few dreams about how the evening would go, many of which turned out to go horribly wrong, and I kept thinking about it during the days leading up to it. But I knew I was going ahead with it and had planned what I would wear and what I would take with me the following week.

I had ticked off anal sex from my sexual bucket list, but now had the opportunity to tick off a threesome.

The night of the dinner arrived and as usual before any date I had gone through the preparatory rituals of hair removal, nails and lashes, exercise and meticulous showering in every orifice.

I had packed a small bag with the essentials (including lube) toothbrush, make up, clean knickers and so forth. In the end I didn't need the lube as Giovanni had loads of it.

When I arrived at his house he had obviously gone to a lot of trouble and laid out an amazing spread of meats, olives and cheeses. He had made gorgeous cannelloni and he had even picked and stuffed some dessert apples from his garden. We were intending to have them for our pudding but never got around to them, rather disappointingly, as they looked really delicious.

After about twenty minutes Francesco arrived with champagne. The lights were low and music easy. Marco had a huge couch in his living room which had soft throws laid over it. It was warm in the house. Everything was set to make me as relaxed as possible. Shortly after dinner somehow the time felt right and the seduction began. Francesco got up from his chair and came to my side to top up my glass. He bent over to kiss me, and at the same time I could see the smile on Giovanni's face as if to give his approval. Francesco and Giovanni took it in turns to kiss me and undress me slowly. They were both very attentive and seemed to enjoy watching each other arouse me and play with me. I felt completely relaxed and knew I would have done anything they had asked me to. Without going into explicit details, when the time was right and I was astride Francesco, Marco entered me from behind. I did tick off another big item from that bucket list. Double penetration. It wasn't something I would ever want to do again but I certainly don't regret it. In fact it was an amazing night. I knew what I was doing and the Italians were fantastic company, and very experienced in their seduction.

I did see the Italians independently again on the following evening, but strangely their magic had gone and I felt I didn't want to get deeper into their world. They had both suggested I join "Killing Kittens" and they wanted me to take them to a Killing Kitten Party.

Killing Kittens is a London-based events company with about 70,000 members, hosting parties designed to sexually liberate women, men and couples. The company is supposedly fully focused on the pursuit of female pleasure for girls in control who know what they want.

Perhaps that was my issue; I didn't really know what I wanted. At the parties, women must approach men, which supposedly keeps "kitties" safe and in control, whilst empowering them to a level of sexual confidence like no other. Guys are the guests.

Francesco and Giovanni wanted me to join Killing Kittens because the association is for women only, and men must be invited by a member. They wanted me to invite them to a party, with the idea, I am sure, of having plenty more threesomes. This never happened and my time spent with these Italian lovers was short.

So what next for me I thought.

Ah yes, the Egyptian. Ludim. He was some sort of shipping mogul. Ludim had a huge flat in Canary Wharf that he had lavishly furnished with extremely expensive Egyptian furniture that was really dark and ugly, and didn't fit the modern space at all.

Again I had met him through Happn.

He invited to me to have dinner at very nice restaurant near St Pancras called Plum and Spilt Milk. This restaurant is in the Great Northern Hotel where I used to meet Marco. Nice choice, I thought. That night, as nearly every night I saw him, he bought the most expensive champagne to drink. I was actually only mildly impressed because

I wasn't even sure if I liked him, and the champagne wasn't really that good either.

Ludim also had a really disgusting habit of smoking these horrible small cigars. I think they were Davidoff Demi-Tasse Cigarillos. Horrible little smelly things and much more toxic than cigarettes. How on earth did I even kiss him? I am not sure why I even met him more than once. Perhaps this was because I was lonely, and maybe because he insisted he bought everything. It was Christmas time and I just did not want to be on my own. We went to dinner on three occasions and I was grateful that we did no more than kiss goodbye as I did not really want to go to bed with him. He said he was a gentleman.

On the third date he asked me if I would like to go away for New Year's Eve. He said we could celebrate in style together. Very randomly, though, he had picked Liverpool as the destination. Why Liverpool, I thought? Why not somewhere exotic? I had nothing else on for New Year so agreed to go with him without really knowing very much about him at all. My kids did not try to talk me out of going, but instead decided it was the perfect opportunity to have a party in my house whilst I was away. I agreed to that, too – and very nearly regretted both my decisions.

Ludim and I did travel first class to Liverpool and it was a lovely hotel. Strong coffee and wine made it just about bearable to kiss him even though I didn't really know why I was there with this man. We did sleep together but the only thing I really remember about that was whilst we were in bed for the first time he let me know that if we were to have any kind of long term relationship my breast implants would have to go. What a nerve. It's pretty bloody obvious to anyone meeting me that my boobs have been surgically enhanced, and if he, or any man, wanted me, then they would have to have me with my implants, or not at all. I kept my feelings to myself, even though I should have punched him.

Our short trip to Liverpool wasn't all a disaster, though. Ludim took me shopping as he said he wanted to buy his sister something nice. He asked me to pick what I think she might like, which I did, but then he gave it straight to me. A beautiful and very expensive Hermes handbag. And he also bought me a bottle of Hermes 24 perfume. I did feel a little like a high class prostitute, which was not the first time I had felt like that, but Hey Ho! the bag was fantastic. And it compensated for that vile breath I had to endure for the weekend.

I never saw this man again, thankfully, which was my choice, but also partly because he went on radio silence after we got back. He said that he had to fly out somewhere to sort some big shipping problem out, but I knew he hadn't even left the country because I was able to tell we had crossed paths again via the Happn app! He did try to contact me once more, but this time I was the one who maintained radio silence until he didn't bother trying any more.

When I returned from Liverpool a little earlier than my kids had expected on New Year's Day, to say that the house looked like a bomb had exploded inside it was a bit of an understatement. Empty bottles, half empty bottles and half empty glasses, bits of unrecognizable food on the table, on the furniture, in the furniture, on the floor, on the walls, on the beds, in the beds.

And it smelt really, really horrible. At least most of the smoking had been in the garden judging by the hundreds of fag butts strewn all over the ground. But to be fair my daughter was furiously tidying up when I arrived, and did point out that I had arrived early without any prior warning. Fair cop I guess. I didn't find anyone asleep in my bed so I couldn't really complain too much. And after all, I had a hideously expensive handbag and some gorgeous perfume so all was not lost.

The item I ticked off next was my "50 Shades" experience as I like to call it. A doctor, and this time about five years older than me.

Keith was charming. Tall, grey haired and very distinguished looking. He was very polite and dressed immaculately in expensive, nice suits. But, like a lot of the men I met he was also married. He always said he wanted to divorce his wife but couldn't bear leaving the two million pound, old house and barn he loved so much, and had put his heart and soul into renovating. The fact that he was another man who was married nearly stopped me seeing him, but he insisted that he was married in name only and his charm offensive won me over as we drove out to have dinner in his gorgeous classic Porsche 911. Keith liked to play games. And he liked to control things in and out of the bedroom.

On one of our evening out dates I was wearing a fairly short skirt and he told me to take my knickers off in the loo in between courses. I thought he was joking but he seemed to have a power over me to make me do things I would not ordinarily do. He looked at me said that I needed to do what I was told if I wanted to please him. I did want to please him and did what he had asked me to do. I sat back down next to him at the dinner table so he could reach underneath it in order to touch me. I don't know why but I let him do it. He even licked his fingers after and said quite loudly, "that was delicious darling". To my relief I don't think any other dinner guests knew what we were doing, but I think the waiter may have guessed.

Because Keith was married sex was always in hotels. He usually gave me instructions as to what he would like me to wear. He didn't like padded bras or stockings with thick tops. He also liked to spank his women. This was not something I had ever tried before. He would make me bend over his knees as he sat down and slap my bottom just hard enough to make the skin tingle but not enough to make me cry. It would turn him on a lot. I wondered why I let him do this but I suppose it was to try out something new, and it seemed harmless enough. It didn't turn me on at all and I could never understand this supposed fine line relationship between pleasure and pain. It was more pain than pleasure in my opinion.

One night as we had sex, he grabbed me by the throat and I could barely breathe. He said this would intensify my orgasm – which I was clearly in no danger of having. He finally released me when he climaxed. In the morning I had huge bags under my eyes and a bruise line around my neck, I never saw him again. Whilst my relationship with Keith did not turn out that well, I know that other couples do enjoy this kind of sexual play.

BDSM – which I think this could be classified as, is apparently becoming very popular, at least if the upturn in sales of whips and chains is anything to go by.

BDSM stands for Body/Discipline/Dominance/Submission/Sadism/Masochism

After this "relationship" ended so abruptly I researched a little more around BDSM and found a good article in Cosmopolitan which helped me understand

1. **BDSM stands for Bondage / Discipline / Dominance / Submission / Sadism / Masochism,** and it covers a huge range of tastes and activities, with endless variations.
2. **It's not all *50 Shades of Grey*.** Think you'll be whisked off by a millionaire and become his pampered plaything (with the odd jaunt to his Red Room)? Think again. BDSM is rarely glamorous,

can be messy and if you embark on a relationship that lasts more than a couple of encounters, it can get pretty complicated unless you walk the emotional line carefully.

3. **Submitting doesn't mean being weak.** It's a gift to give up all control, make yourself more vulnerable than most people could ever imagine and offer yourself, body and soul, for someone else's pleasure… And of course, doing so is also a submissive's ultimate pleasure.

4. **Not everyone can be a good dominant, although plenty of people give themselves that title.** A good dom is completely in control and never lets things get out of hand. They can command obedience with a look or a whisper – so much sexier than some aggressive wannabe screaming orders. The right dom will also get to know their sub. He or she will know when and how to push, and how far.

5. **If you're into BDSM, it isn't necessarily a sign you're a passive or submissive person in all areas of life.** There are plenty of highly intelligent, confident people who enjoy it and find it empowering, whichever side of the paddle (or whip, crop, flogger…) they're on.

6. **BDSM doesn't have to involve sex - it can be a purely mental activity.** Mind games, distance challenges and the fascinating mental interaction between dom and sub is a big part of it for some

people. It's also not all about whips, handcuffs and pain. Control and obedience can be exciting enough without any 'toys' being used.

7. **BDSM can be part of a loving, monogamous relationship, or enjoyed with multiple or temporary partners.** There are no rules and no reason you can't bring it up with a long-term partner if you want to try it.
8. **It's possible to enjoy both sides of the spectrum.** Some people are into being both dominant and submissive - they're called "switches". A switch might be a dom with one partner and a sub with another, or a couple might take turns to play each role.
9. **Safe words do exist.** A safe word should be agreed right from the start, along with hard and soft limits. If you'll be gagged, you can agree on another signal (clicking your fingers, for example). Remember you can always say no; the submissive actually has the most power in an interchange, because he or she can call a halt at any time.
10. **BDSM can be dangerous, with real risks involved.** Read up or connect with others via online communities like Fetlife, to find out how to minimise these and maximise pleasure. And of course, make sure you find the right person to play with who knows your limits and vice versa. Safety is key.
11. **There's a lot of talking involved**, from discussing hard and soft limits, to building anticipation by

planning the next encounter and reliving it afterwards (some people call this 'aftercare' and it definitely helps following an intense scene).
12. **It's totally different to what you'd expect.** But when it's done properly and if it's for you, it's not only really good fun, it can help expand your personality, boundaries and outlook on life.

I remain open minded about BDSM and although I might quite enjoy, on occasion, getting very loosely tied up with a silk ribbons to a four poster bed, it is not for me.

Writing this reminds me of the Spaniard, Luis, and one of the dates with him that I really would rather forget. Luis was about my age, average looking, average build and he worked for an insurance company in London. We crossed paths somewhere near Sloane Square, probably at a wine bare there called the Botanist. It was a bar I would frequently meet some of my friends in after work. It's a really bustling bar and great for people watching. Business men and women, and tourists fill the bar whatever night you go there, and it is a great place to have a drink even if it is extremely expensive. After messaging Luis for a couple of weeks he sounded promising. He also sounded fairly normal which, after some of the dates I had had, was quite reassuring. He was single and doing reasonably well at work. He lived in London, in a flat not too far from the Botanist, and although I didn't sleep with Luis on the first date, I had a feeling it might happen on our second. It was a chilly night and I had stupidly high heels on again which didn't help the walk back to his flat after our night spent drinking in the Botanist. Luis had been drinking vodka most of the evening and was getting very drunk. But he was good company and we laughed a lot.

When the bar closed he invited me back to his flat. I thought I was wobbly on my stupid heels, but he seemed to be swaying quite a bit, too. When we got back to his place he got out a bottle of Grey Goose and suggested we have some shots. I gladly obliged to relax myself as he led me into his bedroom. It was then that I saw what was on the chest of drawers by his bed.

The sight took me completely by surprise. A white towel had been draped across it and laid on top were a variety of implements and sex toys including different shaped and different sized vibrators, dildos, butt plugs and some other scary looking things that I didn't even recognize. It looked like a surgeon's operating trolly. I immediately took another shot and said that I hoped he did not intend using all of those on me. I knew at that moment I needed to get out of there but wasn't sure what I could do. I went to the toilet and sat on the loo for a considerable amount of time. When I came out again the funny thing was that he had collapsed on the bed in a drunken stupor. I was going to come out with a pathetic excuse like I had come on my period and didn't feel well (even though I had had a hysterectomy many years before) but in the end I was able to sneak away. Such a relief. I grabbed my coat and slid out the front door as quietly as possible. Although I had missed the last train home, thankfully my daughter was on hand to help, and I stayed at her flat that night. I think that I had had a very lucky escape. Luis was not so normal after all.

The next date I had was with an average looking Englishman called James. I met him, as with most of my dates, through Happn. He may have been average looking, but I found out later he wasn't exactly average. We arranged to meet at the Ham Yard Hotel – an amazing hotel in Soho. It has its own bowling alley, a roof top terrace, a Spa and Gym and even its own theatre. It revolves around a tree-filled garden with a bronze sculpture by an award winning artist called Kit Kemp. It is very close to the Brasserie I met TJ at and I was a bit worried I might bump in to him there. Thankfully I didn't.

When we met I soon realized money was not a problem for James as not only was the venue expensive, but so was the champagne. I didn't know quite what to make of James at first. He certainly wasn't very good looking. About 50 I think, or perhaps a little older. He wasn't particularly tall, nor athletic. He had very thick glasses on and I even think had a bit of a squint. He was, however, immaculately dressed, and he was extraordinary complimentary of me from the minute I walked in. The champagne flowed continuously, and it's amazing how someone who is very mediocre looking can start to look quite acceptable the more glasses of champagne you have to drink.

James lived somewhere in Hertfordshire and said he didn't need to work anymore as he had made a fortune in property development. He had a villa in Portugal and he owned other properties which he rented out in various locations around London. Unlike a lot of the men I had met, he said he was not looking for a one night stand and what he wanted was a proper "girlfriend". This seemed a bit of a strange thing to say right at the start of our date but as the evening wore on and the champagne continued to flow his slightly odd demeanour didn't seem to matter to me.

Following our drinks at Ham Yard we travelled by taxi to his private members club in Hertford Street, Mayfair. I can honestly say the experience was wasted on me, mainly because I was wasted. I know now that this members' bar is probably one of the most exclusive private members clubs in London, maybe even Europe, and it's a place where the rich and famous go. I could have bumped into Beyoncé and Jay Z and would not have noticed. We had a couple of drinks there and then he suggested I go back to his house in the country.

We went by train and as soon as the train left St Pancras I fell asleep. He woke me up when we needed to get out which was a small station somewhere in the countryside. The walk woke me up and thankfully sobered me up, too, as did the sight of this extraordinary grand house with a gated drive and several outbuildings. James said he kept his toys in them which I later found out to be an Aston Martin and a 1200cc Kawasaki motorbike.

He was a volunteer for the Blood Transfusion service and would be on call to ride around anywhere in London taking bloods to wherever it was needed.

I really didn't know what to think when we went inside. His hallway was bigger than my garden and you could have fitted my entire house inside his kitchen. The kitchen really was very impressive, but also very cold, and it looked like it had never been, or hardly ever been, used.

There was every kitchen gadget you could ever need or possibly imagine, and the biggest wine fridge I think I have ever seen.

We sat in the kitchen for a while sharing a bottle of, what was no doubt, expensive red wine. But we were interrupted quite a few times as James took a lot of phone calls that night. He was apologetic but said they were all important calls from his ex-wife. They were trying to coordinate diaries because she wanted to stay in the villa in Portugal at the same time he did. He talked a lot about his ex-wife and his children and I got the impression the divorce was not his idea. He told me that he had multiple mental health issues and something called sexual anorexia – which was a new one on me. Way too much information for me on a first date.

He showed me around some of the house which included a library, a Sauna, a Gym and a swimming pool. The house also had the most impressive winding staircase leading up to a large landing and the bedrooms. I was clearly going to be staying the night but cannot remember exactly what went on. I understood why nothing probably did happen when I realized what his state of mind was. Early in the morning he told me he had had a call and was needed to pick up some blood and take it to another hospital where it was urgently needed. He told me I could take my time getting ready and he would drive me to the station on his return.

I decided to explore and had a good look in the library where there was one shelf filled with sexual help books, including one on sexual anorexia. The definition was, "A physiological state involving loss of sexual appetite either entirely or episodically, based out of an anxiety or other physiological disorder or by extension a dry spell".

A sexual anorexic has a fear of intimacy to the point the person has severe anxiety surrounding sexual activity and intimate relationships. He later said he had a fear of commitment and was sorry but he wasn't ready for a relationship. He said he had a fear of rejection, and just couldn't bear getting in a relationship that might end leaving him with a broken heart.

His marriage breakdown was perhaps the cause of this, but contrary to what he had said about wanting to find a girlfriend, I think he had just said that in some way to try convince himself that he was getting better, which clearly he wasn't. I messaged him a few times after our date, but he didn't respond at first. Eventually he just sent me a text to say he was sorry, but he had a problem which was nothing to do with me. He just couldn't commit to anything.

Anyone would have thought we had been going out for months and not just had one drunken night out together.

During my internet dating years I met so many men that had so many problems. Problems involving sex: men who climaxed too soon, men who couldn't climax at all, men who wanted to have sex but couldn't, men who needed constant reassuring that they were pleasing me – using lines like "come for me baby – come for me baby". How dare they! The biggest turn off in history.

I had men who liked me to dress up and men who like to dress up themselves. One of the surprisingly common themes was the love of stockings; not stockings worn by me, but worn by them.

I once had a date with a guy who just loved the feel of stockings. We were having sex and I was wearing hold ups at the time. Right in the middle of everything, he took hold of one stocking top and peeled it off, only to put it straight back on one of his own legs. It was clearly a massive turn on for him and he groaned with pleasure as he ran his own hands over his stockinged leg.

I didn't say a thing except, "be careful with that. They were expensive stockings!"

I met another guy, Peter, who actually ran an internet stocking supply company. We met via Happn and arranged to meet at the Kings Cross Rotunda, a quirky restaurant overlooking the canal near the station.

We messaged a lot before our date and he sounded like a really nice guy. He directed me to his website and there was so much choice. Stockings of every possible description. Fishnets, lace, printed, striped, transparent, sheer, garter, thigh-highs, compression stockings, open-toed stockings, opaque stockings, seamed stockings, full body stockings (these literally can be like a full body suit), under-cover stockings, scrunched stockings (vile – Nora Batty type and very un-sexy), and a men's tights and stocking range. There was a phase back then of men reclaiming hosiery fashion. Tights for men were/are definitely a thing. Apparently in 2015 Denise Barber, managing director of "Earth's biggest hosiery store in the UK said, "we sell a great many tights to men. About 40% of our business is with men". It sounds bonkers, but it's true. When you think of it, tights were originally meant for men in Tudor times. Men's tights often come with a handy Y-front style opening at the front. Men like how they feel. They like the warmth. The support. Hosiery for Men suggest the following best options-

1. A manly option: Comfort4Men Men's70 Denier Opaque Tights
2. A budget option: Gipsy 60 Denier XL Tights
3. A luxury option: Falke Pure Matt 100 Denier Opaque Tights

Having mentioned some of the benefits of tights, it is the wearing of stockings by men that is perhaps more interesting. Because as I have said, this was very much a sexual turn on and for at least three men I met this was the case. There definitely was more of a fetish element about wearing the stockings.

Peter asked me what stockings I preferred and on our date brought at least a dozen packs of stockings for me which were all fabulous. Unfortunately, the date was not so fabulous. Peter was just so incredibly boring and could not hold a conversation outside of his stocking business, and as he was extremely boring in looks as well as conversation (although being very "nice") I most certainly did not want to meet up with him ever again.

Just to mention here that the man I met who took my stocking off me to wear himself, Sammuel, suffered incredibly bad sleep apnoea. It is a medical condition that I hadn't come across before. So on the night of the stocking incident I was wide awake after the deed - trying to make sense of what had just happened; he just collapsed and fell in to a deep sleep almost immediately. I tried and failed to drift off, too, and found myself looking at Sammuel in his blissful deep sleep. During the night incredibly he would periodically stop breathing for quite long intervals. I watched him as he literally went rigid and held his breath for what really did seem like several minutes. Seriously scary stuff. I thought he had died on more than one occasion. I thought I would need to call an ambulance, but that if I did I would have to remove my stocking from his leg if he was dead. I wouldn't want to embarrass him – or me – in front of the paramedics, although I guess they would have seen much more bizarre things and anyway if he really was dead it wouldn't have mattered anyway.

I sat there looking at Sammuel sleeping and wondered what I really wanted in life. At that point I still didn't know. I think it is worth mentioning here that Sammuel did actually find true love on Tinder and is now married with a beautiful baby boy. I guess he must have got treatment for his sleep apnoea, or at least his wife was able to become accustomed to it.

My next date worthy of a mention in this book was Colin, the naughty Northerner, or probably a better description would be the not quite got his shit together Northerner. Colin worked in the city and was another guy who loved champagne. He was also another guy who was deeply, deeply troubled. He was a divorcee with a young son who he clearly adored. We talked for hours on the phone before we met and actually got on really well. He was intelligent, funny and also quite exciting. He clearly knew a lot of well-known minor celebrities and did a huge amount of charity work including running the London marathon and many others dressed up in some whacky fancy dress costume. I was to find out later that Colin's sister had died a few years ago of ovarian cancer and he just simply could not accept that she was gone. He had loved her so much and had felt powerless when unable to help her. Now, he couldn't commit to having a relationship with anyone for fear that it might go wrong and he would lose someone else who was close to him. This was my theory anyway.

When I met Colin, I wasn't sure if I fancied him or not which was a bit of a disappointment to be honest, as I had had high expectations following our lengthy late night chats on the phone prior to our first date. However, he was a really smooth talker and the champagne and compliments flowed freely. He was quite honest and said that he didn't really know what he wanted in life but that he loved to drink champagne and make love to beautiful women. He wasn't particularly tall but it looked like he had a good body underneath that very expensive suit he was wearing. He had also sent a few photos of himself in the gym with his biceps pumped up, which I guess should have actually been a warning sign. But the more we drank and chatted, the more I liked him and enjoyed his compliments. One thing which was slightly disconcerting was the thought was that he definitely sought out compliments. He asked me if I liked his pictures on his profile page, and did I like his jacket, did I like his eyes; and this need for me to appreciate his appearance also continued in the bedroom. This was I think because Colin had the most unusually shaped cock. The first time I saw it, well actually it was the first time I felt it, it kind of took my breath away a bit. And not particularly in a good way, either.

Colin had, what I later found out, has been described as "The Hammer" The hammer –shaped penis is a cock which starts with a slimmer shaft leading to a wider head. This narrow base widening to a very wide glans, means that gravity makes it more difficult for this type of erect penis to lift skyward on erection. It looks (and feels) like a mushroom with a narrow base stalk. Colin asked me straight out "do you like my cock?" To be honest I wasn't sure but I didn't feel it very kind to say "What the hell is this?" And in all fairness it didn't feel any different once we were having sex. As long as the width of the penis is OK I don't think most women are bothered about how long or what shape a man's cock is.

There are apparently, broadly speaking, seven types of penis shapes:

1. The Pencil. Described as having a long and thin uniform girth with a narrow head. The length can vary but it is very long and usually thinner than average (Not my type to be honest).
2. The Pepper. The pepper is unusually short (3-4 inches) but exceptionally thick along the entire length (never had one of those but think it could have worked).
3. The Cone. This is a cone which has a linear narrowing of the shaft to a pencil tip. Sometimes this is linked to "phimosis" or tightening of the foreskin that is so restrictive it cannot be retracted at all – quite literally constricting normal expansion of the penis head.

4. The Banana. This features a curve to the left or the right, either naturally, or caused by injury. Some men are born with it, or it is acquired. (Peyronie's disease) 7% of all men will experience this at some point in their life, and it is caused by excess scar tissue developing following an injury, which can lead to lateral deformity, or an hour glass shape.
5. The Hammer – as previously described
6. The Sausage - This is by far the most common penis shape and one I am much more familiar with. This is of average thickness and length with a uniform girth along the length and is fairly typical.
7. The Cucumber -This is a thick cock. It is thick all the way along and a decent length. It is thicker than the usual penis and usually in the 5-8 inch bracket. (This may sound desirable, but can make sex difficult – especially anal sex).

Colin and I saw each other a few times after that initial date. He blew hot and cold. Some days he would message me multiple times saying how much he wanted me, and how he wanted to spoil me. On our second date he brought me a present. It wasn't perfume or a gorgeous new hand bag, but a giant blue butt plug. How romantic and what a disappointment. I did however give it a go in the spirit of trying out new things in the bedroom, and it was rather enjoyable.

Colin's slightly split personality continued as he told me one day that he could see us being in a full-blown relationship only to tell me the next, that it was all over. Then the following week he wanted to see me again. I honestly didn't need this kind of messing around, and he clearly didn't know what he really wanted, so I later replied that we should just end things for good. He replied with a torrent of verbal abuse saying how could I possibly do this to him and what a nasty bitch I was. This really did upset me at the time as I began to think he could be dangerous, and as I had sent him an explicit video the week before I worried he might put it on-line. My advice is never, ever send compromising videos of yourself to anyone. I worried about his for many months afterwards and realize how stupid I was to have sent it.

Colin did actually apologize for his text some weeks later, and we had a nice chat when I bumped into him at Kings Cross about a year later.

My next date was with an extremely tall, dark haired, charismatic and handsome man called Simon. He owned an extremely successful print company in Cambridge and clearly was devoting far too much time to running it, leaving him extremely stressed most of the time. He did have a passion for music and played the guitar in a band when he was able to fit in time for rehearsals and gigs. Simon was exceptionally artistic in nature and I found him a very interesting character who intrigued me. When we messaged each other, the messages were long and very carefully thought out. He was clearly very intelligent and had a fantastic command of the English language. His messages were more like poems or short stories, even. With thoughts about love, life and morals contained in them.

I was excited to be meeting him and extremely curious about how he might be in real life, as it were. He asked me to book somewhere that I would like near Paddington, as that was where he would be coming in to London that day. So I researched the restaurants around that area and found somewhere quirky with a good reputation. I chose Darcie & May Green, situated directly outside Paddington Station, overlooking the Grand Union Canal. The restaurant is actually two boats which share a combined fifty meter upper deck overlooking the canal. Really perfect for a summer rendezvous and designed by Sir Peter Blake, the "godfather" of British pop art. I booked Darcie Green for lunch. It turned out to be a very good choice.

I saw Simon walking towards me before he saw me. He was wearing a Keanu Reeves matrix-like long black coat and also a Fedora, making him look even taller than he actually was, skinny black jeans and a white T-Shirt. He very eccentrically kissed my hand when we met which made me giggle and like him even more than I thought I would. I have never had conversations like the ones I had with Simon with anyone else before. Conversations about, quite literally, the meaning of life, filled with colourful language and propositions. Whilst I enjoyed the cold crisp dry white sauvignon blanc that was effortlessly topped up in my glass, he did not actually drink any alcohol at all. He told me that alcohol had once controlled him and took him to a dark world of depression and occasional suicidal thoughts, a world that he never wanted to return to. Fair enough, I thought, and I had huge admiration for him being able to cut something so negative and toxic, both physically and mentally, out of his life.

Although he did not drink alcohol, I found out pretty soon in to our date that he did enjoy eating hash cookies which he made himself and had brought a big bag with him that day. Thoughts of mine included how very much I would like to try some of these cookies, preferably in a more intimate setting. Simon said that he had taken the somewhat of a liberty of booking a hotel for the night and he had done this even before he had met me. He insisted that there was no obligation on my part to accompany him back to his hotel later that evening but that he would welcome my company.

I did not feel obligated, I just felt aroused and even more curious, and with the inhibitions fading, and feeling a warm glow from the wine we made our way back to the hotel together. We continued our conversations and ordered room service of a selection of cheeses and fruit, and some chips. I ordered gin and tonic, and he ordered a bottle of sparkling water, to wash down the hash cookies he had brought along with him.

He warned me that the cookies were quite strong so I only had one whilst he munched his way through quite a quantity. As the evening went on, I think partly due to the effects of the hash and the alcohol, our voices got louder and louder - as did the accompanying laughter. We decided to start playing our favourite dance tunes and he had brought a mini speaker with him which I plugged my iPad into. I'm struggling to remember why on earth I had brought my iPad – but it was probably because I used it for work and was thinking ahead that I may have needed it for the morning.

We took it in turns to play tracks that we liked and each time took it in turns to remove an item of clothing, whilst dancing around the room like children on too many blue smarties. Finally we were both naked and slightly hysterical. The music was getting louder and louder as we giggled and jiggled about and bounced up and down on the bed.

We failed to hear the room phone ring on more than one occasion but finally noticed loud knocks on the hotel room door. Simon grabbed a dressing gown and I turned the music off. The hotel manager was at the door. He was not pleased. He had received several complaints from the neighbouring rooms about the loud music and screams which were making it impossible for the other guests to sleep. It was, I think, at that point around 2am. Ooops. How naughty of us. Oops indeed. But absolutely hilarious and I nearly peed myself with laughter once the rather flustered manager had left under the reassurance that we would be quiet from then on.

I liked Simon because, on the one hand he was extremely intelligent, and we could have conversations on just about anything from politics and religion down to the best way to cook a turkey – and on the other hand he could be completely childish and play knock down ginger (you know the game when you knock on someone's door and run away before the occupants have a chance to answer). Somehow that's a really funny game to play when you are pissed, or high on hash cookies. I'm not so sure that it is quite so hilarious for the poor person whose door has just been knocked on. My brief thing with Simon, though, could never have lasted. For one thing, he lived too far away, and secondly he was committed to building his business up to a point where he could sell it for a huge amount of money and then fuck off around the world for a few years.

He was probably one of a few of my internet dates that I actually enjoyed having sex with. He was the only one I had an orgasm with.

I think it's probably a good time to bring up the "0" word and consider it properly.

"The Big "O" - The orgasm.

The orgasm. Despite finding so many alternate names for vagina and penis there really just aren't so many synonyms for orgasm, which I find surprising – climax, come, ejaculate (both men and women in some cases). Funny, for some reason I thought there might be more. But I digress.

Putting off talking about having orgasms is something women do a fair amount. Perhaps this is because it is such a personal thing for a woman. In so many movies women seem to be able to have orgasms through penetrative sex with hardly any foreplay which just doesn't, at least in my experience, happen in real life. Men, on the other hand, also from my experience, seem to be able to come fairly easily. Usually, providing the right stimulation is there, and to a certain extent the right mood, they can usually come.

There is also, I think, a lot of misconceptions, often by men again, in my experience, that unless you (the woman they are having sex with) have an orgasm, then you cannot possibly be fully enjoying sex. That in some way, if I do not come, it would mean their failure to satisfy me, or maybe there was something not quite right with me.

I think why sex worked with Simon was because he didn't rush me and there were no expectations from him. We were very relaxed in each other's company and happy to talk about what we did and didn't enjoy in the bedroom. I think I wrote before, one of the biggest turn offs for me was guys who would say ridiculous things like "come for me baby". I just hate that! As if it would be for his benefit, anyway!

In my marriage my husband always wanted me to have an orgasm during sex. It became a chore. Instead of being able to enjoy intimacy and touch I recoiled from it because the pressure on me to have an orgasm was just too great. It is even more difficult to climax if you do not love or fancy the person you are with. This is truer for women than men.

I believe you can enjoy sex without having an orgasm. Just because you don't come it doesn't mean you aren't satisfied. Now that the pressure is removed from me I climax more than I ever thought possible, and sometimes I just have fun. It obviously helps that I deeply love and fancy my partner.

During my time internet dating I became quite an expert at faking orgasms. I was actually quite good at it before to be honest, but tried out lots of different ways depending on the man I was with. It wasn't exactly "When Harry met Sally" all of the time, but I knew when to be noisy (although I nearly got into trouble for that once in the House of Commons) when to hold my breath, squeeze my fanny tight, moan quietly, close my eyes, shudder, etc. etc. I think I could probably run lessons now on how to fake an orgasm. Have you ever played that game, "lust or labour" – you have to look at photos of women's faces and decide whether they are having an orgasm, or giving birth? It is surprisingly hard to tell the difference.

But actually if you are in a loving relationship why would you want to fake it?

There are lots of reasons why I wanted to, or did, fake the big O on my dates. These ranged from actually not really wanting to have sex with someone in the first place, so by faking it sex could be over quickly, to simply just being bored and wanting to get things over with quickly anyway. In fact, when I think of it, most of the time I faked it was because actually it was a good way to get things over with. I am sure some of the men would think, "Ok great she's come - how good am I – now I can get on with it". This would sometimes be followed by, "where do you want it baby? All over your tits? In your mouth? Or inside you?" I would always go for inside – not just because I genuinely prefer that but also because sperm is sticky and a bugger to get off. I also used to think there was no way I would swallow so many calories. Actually I know that's a myth but I think swallowing the cum of someone you don't even want to have sex with is a definite no go.

In literature several types of orgasms have been listed including the G-Spot which I do find hard to believe. This is the one you get from a particular spot internally being stimulated from penetrative sex. It is supposedly markedly different to any other type of orgasm. Believe you me I have had a rummage around in there but never found anything particularly pleasurable, I think my G-Spot must be a gone spot. Who knows though, perhaps one day I might find it and have one of those? I do know that I do experience differing intensities of orgasms and what feels like different types. And I also gush on occasion.

This is female ejaculation (not wee) when the stimulation is harder and more direct. All are extremely pleasurable and without going into detail I have an extremely good sex life now I am older and in love with my partner. I think the sex life in my marriage really fucked me up for a long time. I had sex because I had to. It was a way to manage my ex-husband's behaviour towards me and towards our children. I had sex with my internet dates because it was expected. And I could detach how I really felt from the situation. I thought I was in control with these men but actually it was really the other way around.

I feel so much more differently about sex now than I used to. I think I'm very lucky to be in my fifties with the man I love, and to have similar sex drives, enjoying sex/love making when we are both in the mood, with an ease and honesty I never thought possible. Honesty with your partner in the bedroom certainly helps for both of you to enjoy a much richer and rewarding experience.

I did write earlier about getting into trouble for being too noisy in the houses of parliament, so I guess this leads very nicely back to the dates.

Brief encounter of the political kind -

I always have a huge amount of admin to do in my job and often I will settle myself down in a hotel foyer with a nice cup of coffee and spend an hour or two catching up on things before going home, or in between appointments.

Many other likeminded people do the same. And often you will bump into the same people at the same hotel on numerous occasions. I won't tell you what hotel foyer this was, but I did find myself on quite a few occasions bumping into the same man. He was incredibly friendly and offered to buy me a coffee on more than one occasion. If I'm honest, once again he was not really my type at all. Quite skinny and too pushy. But after chatting about what we did for a living I felt extremely curious to know more about him, and as I was in between internet dates my curiosity got the better of me and I thought "why not?" He told me that he was a Member of Parliament (I think he had a well versed chat up line) and that he would very much like to invite me to lunch in the House of Commons. If I was really lucky he would show me his private chambers (I never heard that one before).

After some initial reservations I thought this would be a really interesting experience and an opportunity I definitely could not refuse. This was despite the fact that he wasn't really my type and the worst thing of all was he was a Conservative. I come from a long line of left wing labour supporters. I have always been open minded about dating people who have different views and beliefs to me. For example, I am an atheist but was married to a catholic, I drink but would be happy to go out with someone who is tee-total, I like meat but could date a vegetarian and I also have lots of friends with differing political views to me. But sleeping with an MP of a right wing political persuasion feels somehow very wrong. I need to say sorry, especially to my sister who is extremely left wing and probably will never forgive me for even contemplating having any kind of sexual relationship with a Tory.

On the day we had lunch I met Steven just outside Westminster Tube station. He seemed somehow very full of himself, and looking back on it a little uneasy. He told me I had to pretend to be there to discuss some sort of constituency matter, of what I can't remember, but I was definitely meant to be on my best behaviour. I had to have my bags searched and scanned and he signed me in. The hall we went into was extremely busy and really loud. I remember he pointed out various MPs and that did indeed seem very strange, to be looking into a world you normally see on TV. After we had had a nice lunch and a few glasses of wine, probably a few too many for me on a relatively empty stomach, he took me on a tour behind the scenes. It was fascinating. We were in the lower part of Parliament, The House of Commons which is made up of about 650 elected Members of Parliament, who make our laws, control the government's finances, keep a supposed close eye on government administration and clearly should not be inviting total strangers into their chambers for a snog.

I learnt recently that it is illegal to enter the Houses of Parliament wearing a suit of armour, which is of little relevance here, but it is also illegal to die there, and that was a bit more worrying as Steven got very cross with me as the date went on. I wish I could remember a bit more about this experience but as happened all too often, I had consumed far too much alcohol. I remember the chambers looking smaller than it does on TV, and there was much ornate woodwork and green leather seating. Little things began to make me giggle which clearly was starting to annoy Steven. I followed him into his private chambers which must have been fitted out fairly recently as it was just a normal boring light-oak panelled office; well, two offices really. There was one room for his secretary on the left who he double checked was not there at that time, and his office was on the right. He had a simple desk with a laptop on it and a small sofa at the back of his office. This was also green leather, just like a mini version of the benches in the hall. I wondered how many more women he had taken to his office, or taken on his sofa, perhaps?

I know I do make a very loud drunk at times, and actually can be annoyingly loud even when I am sober. If I get excited about something I know I can be far too loud. It is something I work on very hard not to be, but often I just forget and lose my self-control. Steven was continually shushing me whilst keeping one ear out for the return of his secretary. He went in for a pash and a fumble on his little green sofa, but clearly his mind wasn't on the action as he was worried he might be caught out. After I had yet again made too much noise, he stopped and told me off. He really had a right go at me saying that I needed to be quiet and behave, this being something which I thought was ironical seeing as he brought me back there. At that point this was all that was needed to sober me up. I got up and said to him we should leave it and it was time I went home. I think it was a lucky escape as number one, I didn't fancy him and number two, he was a right-winged little cock.

I did get messages from him after that from time to time but I politely told him I was too busy to meet. I also remember bumping in to him in a restaurant on King's Road where he offered to bring me champagne and chocolates and spend the day in bed. This was never in a month of Sundays going to happen.

So, what's next on the bucket list.

Another item which was ticked off, not via the internet dating route, but just via whispered conversations and someone who knew someone who knew someone that would definitely be in to it. This was the two women one man experience. Another experience which I got to tick off but didn't really go according to plan. A friend of mine who, at the time, knew that I was exploring my sexuality in ways that I didn't quite understand, said I should meet up with this couple she knew of via a friend of hers who were definitely out to have some sexual fun with another interested lady. It turned out they were a doctor and his practice nurse. Dr Dick M and his practice nurse, Beverly, clearly enjoyed a bit of extramarital sex (I found out later that they were both married but not to each other). Somehow phone numbers were exchanged and we made arrangements to meet a couple of weeks later. I have not, and still do not, fancy other women even though of course I can acknowledge and even admire a woman who is beautiful, and has great legs or boobs for example.

I was not entirely sure that I really did want to go through with this meeting but I did think that perhaps if I found a woman attractive then maybe, just maybe, if the circumstances were right and I fancied the man, I could get aroused and maybe enjoy a very different kind of sexual experience. We agreed to meet in a bar in a small hotel in East Sussex. I was very nervous and kept thinking to myself, "what on earth am I doing here? This is just not me". But when they walked in the bar I could see Beverley was very attractive, as was Dr M, and after a few glasses of wine were drunk it was time to go up to the bedroom. We helped each other take off our clothes and Dick gave me a passionate kiss as Beverley looked on. I then watched them as they kissed, after which Beverley approached me. Sadly, although I kissed a girl, unlike Katy Perry, I did not like it.

It was weirdly a bit of a disappointment to be honest. I really wasn't sure what I should do next, but the one thing I did know was I didn't want to continue with this experience. Faking it until you make it was not going to work in these circumstances so I simply had to tell Dick and Beverley that it just wasn't for me. I didn't know how they would react but they were actually very understanding about the whole situation and just said it really wasn't a problem as they were still having a good time. After my admission I filled up their glasses of wine, put them on the bedside table and left them to it.

This short experience taught me that I really needed to be more honest with myself about what I was looking for. I still could not decide what that was.

The following week I messaged my German on and off shag and spent the night in his flat in London enjoying his athleticism - and his frog squatting ability. I also enjoyed his breakfast as he did this fantastic poached egg with crispy bacon on chili, smashed avocado on sour dough thing. Worth staying the night just for the breakfast, if nothing else.

I decided to go back to Happn and have a look at who I might have crossed paths with that week. I had travelled up to London on business quite a bit and felt that I must have brushed past someone interesting.

There was one match that had definitely piqued my interest. His name was Mark and he really was drop-dead gorgeous. The fact that he was drop-dead gorgeous and had liked me should have been a warning sign. He was the owner of a very successful Broadcasting PR Agency based in London, or at least he said he was. I wish I had kept all the details I had of him to warn other unsuspecting women like me. We messaged each other a lot and sent some very steamy photos across. I was careful to avoid sending anything too explicit but I did get a lot of him posing in bed with just the right amount of flesh on show. I don't know why I was so drawn in to the idea of being with this obvious narcissist. It wasn't even the money or the body that got me wanting to meet him; he just had a way of making me feel comfortable and he was really good at flattery without being unbelievable. Our messages turned in to phone calls where he made me laugh, and talked about how we would meet for dinner very soon. He said he had a young son who he loved more than anything in the world, and although separated from his mum he would have him at weekends and whenever he could. He said he was looking after his son for a couple of weeks and then we would meet. Our conversations invariably moved from general chit chat to conversations about what we found attractive in our partners and how we could please each other. I found myself planning what to wear on our first date around what he said he found sexy in a woman. Absolutely no thongs and definitely no padded bras. Incredibly I went out and bought some Bridget Jones knickers. "What the hell," I can almost hear you say. Surely I was confident enough in my own skin to wear the knickers I wanted to – which definitely did not include knickers that my mum would have been wearing. Although on the plus side I have to say they were incredibly comfortable and made a nice change from having a cheese wire stuck up between the cheeks of my arse.

As for the no padded bra, as my boobs are surgically enhanced they do not actually need a lot of lifting and separating so a nice lacey bra worked OK. I just look back now and again I am thinking what on earth was I doing.

We fixed a date to meet and a time for him to pick me up from St Pancras. I made a huge effort to prepare perfectly for our first date and it took me ages to get ready. When I got to the station he was nowhere to be found, and despite numerous phone calls and waiting for over an hour he didn't turn up. I had to simply wait for the next train home feeling completely perplexed. A couple of hours later I had a message from him apologizing profusely, saying he had given me the wrong date and that he had been in a business meeting all night so he couldn't see my missed calls. Although I was disappointed, I believed him and I said it was OK. We fixed another date to meet in the coming weeks. When the day arrived, I messaged to confirm timings for the evening, and spent the afternoon getting ready including choosing which pair of large knickers I was going to seduce him with later.

But once again, when I got to London and waited for him he didn't turn up. This time I wasn't disappointed; I was downright bloody angry. I messaged and called him till I realized he was not going to answer me and then went to the nearest bar to get drunk. I did get one message from him a couple of days later to say that for various reasons he just couldn't go through with meeting me. There wasn't even an apology. I felt incredibly stupid as I had invested so much time, energy and emotion in this potential relationship, even down to thinking about long term possibilities, which sounds absolutely ridiculous, I know, but he was just so damn convincing. I found out a few weeks later, purely by chance, that he had done this to other women. I was chatting to the lady who does my eyelashes and who always loved to hear my internet dating stories and I told her about the gorgeous looking man who had failed to turn up twice despite the endless hours of preparation I had done. I mentioned his fondness for Bridget Jones knickers and unpadded bras. She asked me to show her his profile picture and as soon as she saw it she said she had another client who had been through exactly the same thing with him. Hours of preparation, big knickers and big expectations only to be stood up on the night they were supposed to meet. Her client actually went to meet him three times before she eventually realized he was never going to materialize and finally told him in no certain terms to "stop fucking about with women's lives and go sort your own fucking life out first".

It seems he got something out of being able to manipulate women even without meeting them. I guess he got a kick out of being able to control how a woman dressed and never had any intention of meeting them. I wonder now if the profile pictures and other pictures were real and maybe he had some sort of serious mental or physical condition. Maybe he was a fifty- stone recluse who had never had a real girlfriend. Or perhaps he was, in fact, a she. All kinds of possibilities went through my mind but at least I didn't get financially scammed like some women have been through; "catfish" scams as they are called now.

I did get to actually meet my next date, Tom, in person and he seemed a really normal, nice man. – But – and there always seemed to be at least one but – he was another married man.

Arghhhhhhhhhhhhhhhh. He was Irish and although his home was in Dublin, with his wife and two children, he spent weeks away due to a national sales role. He spent a lot of that time away in London. The usual excuses were made to me that the love had gone from his marriage a long time ago, and they didn't have sex anymore but stayed together for the sake of the children. This story was told to me several times during my dating years and looking back on it I should have just told all of them to fuck right off. Tom was fairly believable in the sense that I really did believe he was stuck in a loveless marriage. He said they had discussed separating on numerous occasions and maybe if either of them found love this is what they agreed to do.

Whilst I wasn't totally convinced of Tom's situation, I did fancy him quite a lot. And after meeting a few times for drinks and having had a really promising kiss I began to think of taking it further.

One week we were both in London for work meetings at the same time and we both had hotel rooms booked. It had seemed pretty obvious to me that we would sleep together one night during that week. So we fixed a day that worked best for both of us. I made my preparations as usual, including removing every bit of unwanted hair down to the very last follicle. After we had had a few drinks at the hotel bar I was staying in, we got a bottle of nice bubbly and took it up to my room. There was much kissing as you would imagine, inevitably leading to taking off each other's clothes and the atmosphere was electric. I unbuttoned his shirt and began to take it off, feeling his chest with my fingers, slowly caressing his… well, what was I caressing? I was completely horrified and taken utterly by surprise by what felt like the fur of a very, hairy mountain gorilla! This was not just any old hairy chest, and as a matter of fact I really like a soft, hairy chest. No. This was the hairiest chest I have ever had the unfortunate experience to get up close to. Thick, coarse, long black hair that covered every square centimetre of his chest, and indeed his entire body. I didn't know quite what to do. Suddenly all the passion I had been feeling completely evaporated.

What would you have done in those circumstances? Would you have faked how you really felt and admired the warm, hairy, thick nest that seemed to be part of his torso, or somehow would you find a way to make the whole excruciating experience stop. As much as I had had sex with someone before who I really didn't want to, at least they had always been human. If this guy had had a beard he literally could have been mistaken for something that had escaped from London Zoo. I had to think very quickly, and to give myself a chance, I retracted my hand from the tangled web of his chest and said I suddenly was desperate from the loo and had a very bad stomach cramp.

I locked myself in the loo and messaged my eldest to say that she had to call me in the next minute without fail, no matter what she was doing, or I was at grave risk of committing bestiality. Thank god she answered, although the reply was, "WTF mum? What have you done now?"

Sure enough about thirty seconds later she called me. I walked out of the bathroom holding the phone to my ear (meanwhile the ape had undressed and was already lying back in my bed, trying to look sexy with a glass of bubbly in hand. I half expected him to make some sort of mating call).

"Oh my God, darling. Are you OK?" I screamed down the phone." Yes, of course I'll come right away. Your poor thing". I told Tom that my daughter was bawling her eyes out down the phone as she had split up with her boyfriend, and managed to crash her car on her way home from work.

We would have to postpone our jungle romp until another day – so sorry. I needed to be with her.

Tom, although disappointed, was remarkably understanding, even offering to come with me. I virtually pushed him out of my bedroom as soon as he was dressed and necked the remaining champagne. To complete my deception, I got dressed and left the hotel in case he was watching. I have looked back at this experience and considered that I must have been really shallow. How could I possibly have rejected this man simply because he was hairy? And then I remember more clearly that he wasn't just hairy, he was in fact, a gorilla. And I am relieved that I didn't go through with things. I am certain that if I had I would have been scarred for life.

He didn't really understand why I kept putting him off when he repeatedly asked if we could meet another time. The following week he went back to Ireland and then eventually he stopped messaging me when he realized I was no longer interested.

I was starting to think this dating madness was just utterly pointless and that I would never find anyone I could be honest with; be my true self with. However, despite all the lost causes and near misses I was still not entirely disillusioned. I remained hopelessly optimistic and I continued to use my Happn app, and intermittent Tinder dates, many of which invariably proved a complete waste of time. More dick pics and more rather dodgy profiles. Men who turned up and were disappointingly shorter than they said they were, or were several sizes larger than they had appeared to be on their profile pictures. Men who definitely were older than they had stated on their profile pages, or in many cases they just seemed completely weird. I would definitely suggest that you do not agree to meet a man whose profile picture is a motorbike, a dog or a packet of Marlboro lights. Enough said.

Following my encounter with an escapee from London Zoo, I crossed paths with Steven. He looked relatively normal from his photographs on his profile page.

He wasn't earth-movingly handsome, but then again, he wasn't someone I would turn around and walk in the opposite direction from, either. He was about the right age and a clearly successful businessman, working in the City. He rented a flat in Canary Wharf and owned a gorgeous converted barn in East Sussex. His working hours were so long that he rented the flat in London during the week and stayed in his barn over the weekend. To me this sounded very promising indeed. We messaged quite a few times and I learnt that he was single. HURRAH. He had a teenage son who was in boarding school during term time, but stayed with him on various holidays. Steven was a Manchester United fan but I couldn't really hold that against him. We messaged quite a bit but then finally spoke in person to arrange our first date. He had a nice calm, soothing voice. I began to get my hopes up, and felt quite excited about meeting him. It was a cold winter and we had had a few flurries of snow, some of which had settled. I am looking out my window as I write this and the rain is yet again torrential, with gusts of wind topping 60 miles per hour or more. Storm Ciara and Storm Dennis have really taken their toll in the UK and I am sick of it. Writing on this date just brings back memories of how wonderful the weather was on the day I met Steven. There wasn't a cloud in the sky, which seemed ultra-blue and the countryside simply looked so picturesque. We had decided to meet for a walk in the local forest and the plan was to build up an appetite for a nice pub lunch. This was such a contrast to all the other first dates I had had which were almost always in a bar in London. When we met I was slightly disappointed to find that although facially Steven was almost as I had expected, he was very much bigger than his profile picture had led me to believe. He said, very honestly, that he really needed to get exercising a bit more and drink less red wine, but he had been incredibly busy at work and had let things go.

I decided that I should just try not to be so judgmental and despite the few extra spare tyres he had a warm smile, and was a good conversationalist. I really thought that as long as he wasn't covered in a blanket of dark coarse hairs I might just be able to fancy him. The walk in the forest was surprisingly enjoyable. We seemed to get on really well and I decided that perhaps this might actually work. He spoke thoughtfully and was flattering in just about the right amount. He said that he was relatively new to the dating scene having been divorced for only a few months. He said he had not had the nerve to start seeing anyone until recently. We didn't have sex on the first date. Firstly, it may have been because it was day time and I hadn't had time to make the necessary preparations. Those being the obligatory shaving of the pubes and ensuing I had on my matching underwear. Also, after a large roast dinner I was carrying a rather huge food-baby around with me. Even though he was quite chubby I really didn't want him to see my stomach bulging over slightly old knickers, and the other slight worry I had was there was always a risk of me letting out a particularly smelly fart after all the red cabbage I could not resist eating at lunch. Following our first meeting we arranged a second date which was to be at a pub near his barn the following weekend.

Steven knew I had an incredibly challenging and busy work week ahead of me and I was utterly delighted that the next afternoon a bunch of flowers was delivered to my house with a note to wish me a good week ahead and that he was very happy that we had met. Wow. That made me stupidly happy. Stupidly.

The next time me met I was understandably perfectly prepared. I was wearing matching underwear and there was certainly not a chance of a fart in earshot as I hadn't eaten very much that day at all. I knew I was in danger of getting a little too tiddly a little too soon but due to my lack of self-control this didn't stop the first large cold glass of pinot slipping down far too easily.

We had a good evening and as I had expected we did go back to his converted barn together. What a beautiful building it was, too. There was a large open plan living space with a log fire and several extraordinarily comfortable sofas. Everything about the place suggested money was not a problem and I couldn't help but be impressed by the quality of all the fixtures and fittings. Whilst I can appreciate all that money can buy I am really not impressed by someone just because they have money. I can admire beautiful things, enjoy staying in beautiful places and enjoy expensive food and wine, but I don't get envious of people who have money, whether they have worked hard for it, or not. I know first-hand that money doesn't bring you happiness.

Having said all that, I wouldn't have minded living in that barn; it really was spectacular.

We went to bed that night and the sex was OK, I suppose. It was neither earth shatteringly orgasmic nor completely dreadful either. After that night we saw each other a few times and I thought we had had a pretty good time. I even began to think that things might start going somewhere. The sex was never memorable but he never seemed to complain. And then the messages just fizzled out. Steven would send me the odd, rather boring message and occasionally would suggest times to meet, only to cancel things at short notice. I got the feeling that he was no longer interested in me and that it was time to end things. Eventually I messaged him to let him know how I felt. He did reply to say that he was sorry I felt that way, and he tried to explain why he wasn't ready for anything serious. He pretty much admitted that as he was so new to the dating scene following his divorce that he wanted to go and meet new women and try new things before he would consider being in a relationship again. I can't really blame him as I was in similar circumstances a few years before when I had just divorced. What he really wanted to do was play the field and have some fun. Rather strangely he contacted me out of the blue not that long ago to say he had made a mistake and really wanted to see me again.

I was really pleasant to him and even said if we were ever in London at the same time I would be happy to have a coffee and catch up. I told him that I was in a committed relationship now and very happy. He then started sending me really smutty messages which were very explicit and seemed really out of character. I had to block him in the end which made me think I had had a lucky escape.

After Steven I really thought I was done with internet dating and that I should just leave things to chance. I was going to delete all the contacts I had made through Happn but accepted one more invite out to dinner with Marco, the young Italian I had met many months before. I had already told him that I didn't want to see him again. I had explained that I couldn't see us in a long term relationship and this was what I was starting to yearn for. Marco was, after all, much younger than me, and had said that he wasn't ready to commit to anything serious. But he was single and he was persuasive, saying that he had had a promotion at work and really wanted to celebrate with me.

His charm and persuasive nature paid off and I agreed to meet him in London to celebrate his success. Just one last night I said to myself as I began my preparations. This was to be the last time I would see him. In fact it was to be the last time I went out with anyone for some time.

We met at a hotel bar close to St Pancras. I just did not feel right that night and I was feeling like I was in someone else's body. I felt as if I was on a kind of auto-pilot. I knew in my head that actually I didn't really want to be at the bar, drinking champagne with a man I knew would only ever be an occasional date when it suited him. But somehow I played the part that was expected. Wearing the right clothes, saying the right things, laughing suggestively at the right moments. And following him up to his room when he wanted to go to bed. My head was spinning as we undressed. The hotel room was small but very plush. The bed had piles of silky pillows and above the headboard was a huge gold edged mirror. It wasn't long before he turned me over to take me from behind. I didn't want anal sex but for some reason I just went along with it. And during the act he told me to look up at the mirror to watch. He shouted out fairly loudly, "Oh my god. It's like I'm in a porn movie". But I didn't want to be in a porn movie. I didn't want to play a part any more. Those words really affected me that night and that was the moment that I realized I simply did not want to be doing this anymore. I thought I had been in control but had to be honest with myself that this had never really been the case. I had been with men that I really didn't want to be with and I had been pretending to myself that it was making me happy.

In fairness, at the start, maybe it did. I really didn't want a relationship after I split up with my husband, and I wanted to explore sex with a freedom I had not had before.

I don't regret most of what I did, and I did have some fun, but the time had come for me to just enjoy being single and realize I could enjoy my own company. I was certain that I would never find a man that loved me for who I really am. Someone who I could truly call my soulmate. A man I could laugh with, enjoy being a couch potato with whilst watching the football on Sunday afternoons. A man that loved me despite my flawed skin, imperfect body and annoying habit of talking far too loudly, especially when drunk.

For a while I was content with my own company. I enjoyed binge watching box sets on TV and eating microwave dinners (I can recommend a tasty Waitrose prawn linguini) washed down with a nice cold bottle of Sauvignon Blanc. It's quite funny really; I got by very happily without ever turning my oven on and it was only when I invited my current partner over for dinner for the first time, I realized I didn't even know how to turn it on. In truth I ended up asking my son how to do it.

Last weekend I surprised our friends by actually cooking something from scratch. I made everything including the sauce for my Italian Stallion Sausage Casserole to the Chocolate Butterflies for the Pots au Chocolat dessert. I had to take pictures during the cooking to prove to my friends I had done it all rather than just buy it ready made, and take it out of the containers to look like I had done it– something I had done several times before.

Chapter 9

A Happy Ending?

I smile as I come nearer to the end of my story as far as this book goes. The beginning of my story for me really starts when I met my soon-to-be husband, surprisingly, on Tinder.

I had sworn off internet dating but I was beginning to feel lonely again and my eldest daughter convinced me just to take one more look at a few more Tinder profiles.

I looked at a few and instantly swiped left knowing they would not be right for me. I was literally whizzing through them whilst watching another episode of Homeland when one profile made me stop. And he had "super" liked me. I stopped because there was the photo of a man who looked somehow like he would be really kind. He just had the look of a man who would be nice to me. I cannot quite explain why I got this feeling. Maybe it was the lack of staged photos or the fact that he had these eyes that just seemed to suggest he had been hurt himself and wanted a partner that he could trust. I questioned whether I was simply making this all up, and in all honesty I probably was. Except that for once my instinct turned out to be right.

We messaged each other quite a bit before we actually met, and because I would like this final chapter of my story to remain private, at least to some extent, I am not going to go into any intimate details.

I can say that he genuinely is the best thing that ever happened to me and I feel extraordinarily lucky after everything I have been through to finally find a man I am truly and deeply in love with. And it turns out he also had been through tough times: redundancies, difficult divorce, bereavement and infidelity to name but a few.

We are a couple who are not perfect. We don't agree on everything and we certainly don't support the same football team. But we laugh so much together and support each other unconditionally and we know we want to grow old – or rather grow older – together.

By the time this book is published we will be married and we will no doubt be enjoying a large glass of cold, crisp, dry wine together, laughing or shouting at the telly, depending on which football team is winning. We will be drunk and shopping off Amazon together and then be surprised when a table gets delivered the next day and we can't even remember ordering it. We will decide we can't be bothered cooking so just get a nice French stick, cheese and pate to nibble in front of the TV.

He will tell me I am beautiful when I have a new spot erupt, and he will mean it. I will tell him he has the best bum, and I will mean it.

P.S

I hate getting old. And I hate that I am so obsessed about it. But I know I can deal with it now. I am always going to try out the latest skin cream that claims to have incredible rejuvenating properties, and buy the latest foundation to make my skin look flawless, only to find out it really doesn't. But I can now laugh about it with my partner and it is all becoming so less important.

I wish all those who have read this book a happy and healthy future. And if you are someone who is looking for love then please don't give up. Don't be afraid to do something outside your comfort zone; you never quite know where it will take you.

And my message to you as Bob Marley once sang, "Don't worry about a thing. 'Cos every little thing is going to be alright"

P.P.S

COVID 19 and stealth shagging

I was not going to write anything about the dreadful situation that we all now find ourselves in. I wanted to end this book on a high. But the outbreak of Coronavirus has been devastating to so many people and I do not know how things will turn out. There will be books, films and the inevitable Netflix series I am sure. During lockdown everyone has had to find ways of coping.

Something that has made me giggle though and I thought worth a mention was "stealth shagging" as we are now calling it.

As there are currently four adults living in our house, two of whom are my children, it can sometimes be very difficult to get any time to be intimate with my partner. Un-deterred though, as soon as I have persuaded the children take the dogs out together, and as long as we are both in the mood, stealth shagging can commence. We pause the TV, rush upstairs for a quick one, get dressed, comeback down and restart the programme where we left off. The kids return, not exactly unsurprised, to see us watching the same programme, but with perhaps the jumper I was wearing before they left, on back to front, a red face and a guilty looking smile......

Some useful websites-

BEAT- the UKs Eating Disorder Charity – www.beatingdisorders.org.uk

Mind – the mental health charity for all types of mental health problems – www.mind.org.uk

Helpline – Eating Disorders Support – www.eatingdisorderssipport.co.uk

Getting a divorce – www.citizensadvice.org.uk

Divorce advice/Family Lives – www.familylives.org.uk

British Association of Dermatologists help with skin problems both emotional and physical – www.skinsupport.org.uk

Help-lines

-Beat – (eating disorders) 0808 801 0677
www.beatingdisorders.org.uk
email: help@beatingdisorders.org.uk

-Anorexia & Bulimia Care (ABC) 0300 11 12 13
www.anorexiabulimiacare.org.uk

-Help line – Eating disorders support
Tel 01494 793 223

Samaritans – 116 123

NHS 111

Random photos –

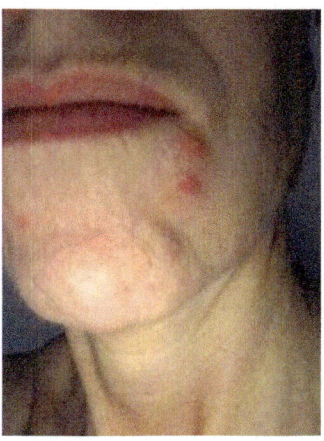

Even at fifty I was still plagued with skin problems – from the trip to Milan

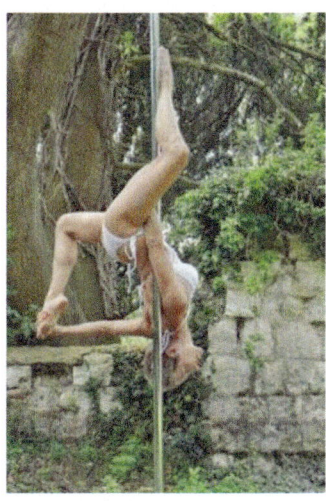

I can't do this anymore – but it was fun whilst it lasted!

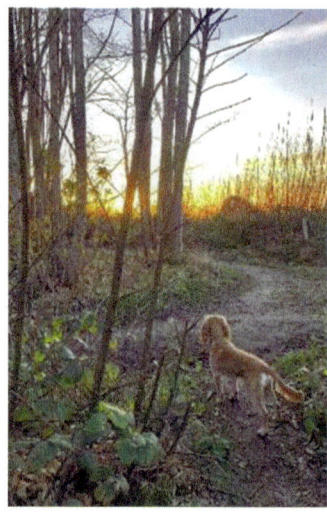

A walk with my dogs in these beautiful woods never fails to cheer me up

Printed in Great Britain
by Amazon